OVERVIEW-MAP KEY

RECOMMENDED RIDES

Rides with 2,001 to 3,000 Feet of Climbing

Rides with More Than 3,000 Feet of Climbing

Rides with Jumps

Rides with Extreme Drops

Rides with Shuttles

Lonely Rides

Crowded Rides

MOUNTAIN BIKE!

LOS ANGELES COUNTY

CHARLES FALK PATTERSON

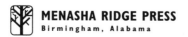
MENASHA RIDGE PRESS
Birmingham, Alabama

DISCLAIMER

This book is meant only as a guide to select trails within and around Los Angeles County and does not guarantee rider safety in any way—you ride at your own risk. Neither Menasha Ridge Press nor Charles Patterson is liable for property loss or damage, personal injury, or death that may result from accessing or riding the trails described. Be cautious when riding on or near boulders, steep inclines, and drop-offs, and do not attempt to explore terrain that may be beyond your abilities. To help ensure an uneventful ride, please read carefully the introduction to this book. Acquaint yourself thoroughly with the areas you intend to visit before venturing out. Ask questions and prepare for the unforeseen. Familiarize yourself with current weather reports, maps of the area you intend to visit, and any applicable trail regulations.

Copyright © 2008 by Charles Falk Patterson
All rights reserved
Published by Menasha Ridge Press
Printed in the United States of America
Distributed by Publishers Group West
First edition, first printing

Cover design by Travis Bryant
Text design by Steveco International
Cover and interior photography by Charles Falk Patterson
Author photograph by Stephanie Kalinowski
Cartography and elevation profiles by Charles Falk Patterson, Scott McGrew, and
    Lohnes+Wright
Indexing by Galen Schroeder

Library of Congress Cataloging-in-Publication Data

Patterson, Charles Falk.
Mountain bike! Los Angeles County/Charles Falk Patterson.
    p. cm.
  ISBN 13: 978-0-89732-646-9 (alk. paper)
  ISBN 10: 0-89732-646-6 (alk. paper)
  1. All-terrain cycling—California—Los Angeles County—Guidebooks. 2. Los Angeles
County (Calif.)—Guidebooks. I. Title.
  GV1045.5.C22P6763 2007
  796.6309794'93—dc22
                              2007006396

Menasha Ridge Press
P.O. Box 43673
Birmingham, Alabama 35243
www.menasharidge.com

TABLE OF CONTENTS

For Kye, Casey, Michael, John, and Mary
—*C. F. P.*

ACKNOWLEDGMENTS

First and foremost, I'd like to thank fate for allowing me to complete roughly 200,000 feet of ascending and descending more than 500 miles without crashing or crossing paths with mountain lions, landslides, runaway trucks, Africanized bees, rabid bison, or mosquitoes tainted with West Nile virus. Fate also canceled Stephanie Kalinowski's early meeting with her maker, providing enough bushes for her to grab as she fell down one of Lower Sam Merrill Trail's many slides, averting catastrophe. For that, Stephanie and I are truly grateful.

I extend warm thanks to the many persons whose brains I picked along the way, among them Kye Sharp, Casey Kelley, Deker Williams, Michael Kelley, and Mike Stanosek.

The staff of Helen's Cycles Westwood served as my pit crew—keeping me properly outfitted and listening to my stories all the way through. I dread the day when the managers, Mike "Fukazaki" Feng and Pete Burnham, move on to bigger and better things. El Maestro Mecánico Gilberto Quintanella kept my bike from missing a shift the whole way—¡Muchas gracias, señor! Special thanks to Ryan Morse for building me a pimp set of wheels and for all the laughs.

Thanks to Patrick Rose, Maria Biber-Ferro, Quito Cooksey, Deker Williams, Gabriela Williams, Jason Tuttle, and Stephanie Kalinowski for making great riding buddies, photographers, and photographic subjects.

Perhaps the biggest thank you should go to the volunteer workers and park employees who have done such a fantastic job of maintaining the trails of Southern California. Without their tireless efforts, the forces of nature would surely take away many of our greatest trails within just a few seasons. Thanks, guys and gals, your work is much appreciated!

ABOUT THE AUTHOR

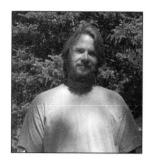 **Charles Falk Patterson** grew up in Topanga Canyon, California, the ideal place to become an avid mountain biker. If the local trails weren't inspiring enough, Charles found additional motivation from his mother, Casey, and brother, Kye, both former professional racers. Being neither an insanely fast downhiller like his brother nor possessing the masochistic level of endurance that his mother used to win RAAM (Race Across America) in 1987, Charles would have ride just for fun until Menasha Ridge Press gave him the opportunity to write this book and leave his own mark on the sport. Very much addicted to all forms of two-wheeled locomotion, Charles hopes to keep hammering the cranks and twisting the throttle long after he's eligible for senior discounts and Social Security checks.

PREFACE

Mountain biking has changed a great deal since its inception roughly 30 years ago. What was once a small group of pioneers getting together for some fat-tire fun in the woods has now become a massive, multifaceted sport of several disciplines. On the competitive side, you can now race single-speed, cross-country, downhill, 24-hour, dual slalom, super-D, mountain-cross, and freeride. Each discipline has a unique following of riders who use specialized equipment and preparation to compete in their field.

The evolution of these disciplines has created an unfortunate rift between the two largest groups—the downhillers and the cross-country crowd. In many ways, this is a battle of young against old. The general gripe from the cross-country set is that the young downhill punks are destroying the trails, not observing proper trail etiquette, scaring equestrians and hikers, and causing, through their careless antics, the closure of public lands. From my perspective—being neither one nor the other—I have noticed that, although there are a few careless downhillers out there, the cross-country riders are just as guilty of the aforementioned sins. The issues mentioned above—etiquette, trail erosion, and colliding with other trail users—have been hot topics since bikes had no suspension and today's downhillers were nothing more than unfertilized eggs. The simple truth is that all mountain bikers, whether wearing spandex or baggies, riding ultralight hardtails or long-travel freeride bikes, can be guilty of these crimes.

When I got the opportunity to contribute to this trail guide, I wanted to address a weakness I perceived common to other trail guides on the market: I believe a lot of them spoke only to riders of the cross-country set, neglecting the diversity of the sport. Whether you live for the climb or the descent, I want you to feel as if this book was written for you.

I knew prior to getting started that the mountain biking in and around Los Angeles County is superb, but I learned along the way that it is more than that. Los Angeles is, perhaps, the perfect place to live if you're a mountain biker. Every imaginable type of terrain, for every type of rider, is accessible from the area. I know this statement could spark protest from residents of other world-class mountain biking areas like British Columbia, Northern California, and Southern Utah. What I feel gives Southern California the edge over those places and others is the weather. Where else can you find such great riding terrain with such agreeable weather? We get to ride year-round. What more can you ask for?

What also makes Los Angeles County such an ideal mountain biking locale is that it has two mountain ranges—the Santa Monicas and the San Gabriels, which cater to two distinct mountain bike personalities. The Santa Monica Mountains, arguably the mellower of the two ranges, have plenty of options for the cross-country rider who prefers climbing to navigating technically challenging terrain. The Santa Monicas, being milder, are great for newcomers to the sport because the rides are generally less steep, dangerous, and technical than those of other areas.

The San Gabriel Mountains, in the Angeles National Forest, are great for the more adventurous, experienced, extreme rider who favors action over calorie burning (although calories will be burned in either range). The trails of the San Gabriels are truly underrated and underappreciated by residents of Southern California and the mountain biking community as a whole. I'm surprised, after covering almost everything the LA area has to offer, how little your average SoCal mountain biker knows about the San Gabriels.

If for any reason you find your mountain biking personality out of place in these mountain ranges, just take a leisurely boat ride to enjoy the enchanted, windswept roads of Catalina Island. If that's not enough, take a road trip to the Los Padres National Forest to tread the pine-needle-crusted trails of Mount Pinos. Or drive a little farther and savor the high-desert scenery of the Alabama Hills below Mount Whitney. With so many different environments to choose from year-round, Southern California truly is the best place to ride mountain bikes, and Los Angeles County is the epicenter.

This trail guide is made up of mostly well-known trails and a few lesser-known routes that, to my knowledge, have never been included in any previously published trail guide for mountain bikers. Generally, my routes favor technical riding and singletrack for the descent, reserving wide fire roads and pavement (if any) for the climb. I believe most mountain bikers would have it this way. For the rare biker who prefers technical climbs and would rather take the fastest, easiest, most direct route down: I encourage you to just ride my routes backward.

I have also attempted to minimize the number of miles spent on wide, groomed dirt roads and paved roads. This isn't a trail guide for roadies or cyclo-crossers. This guide is for riders of 26- or 29-inch-wheeled, fat-tired, off-road bicycles who seek technical, off-road terrain. In a perfect world, every route in this book would be 100 percent singletrack, but that's not the case because there simply aren't enough legal multiuse singletracks in and around Los Angeles County to make that possible. Despite this, you may find, as I have, that a long, secluded pavement ascent is a blissful experience and a groomed fire-road descent can be a slice of heaven.

Mountain bikes are all-terrain, human-powered vehicles that can take you anywhere. Unlike gas-powered vehicles and horses, mountain bikes don't require gasoline, hay, or words of encouragement to keep moving. What other form of all-terrain transport can be thrown over your back and carried to safety? Southern California is the ideal environment to explore with the ideal form of wilderness locomotion—the mountain bike. I hope this is the ideal guide.

—*Charles Falk Patterson*

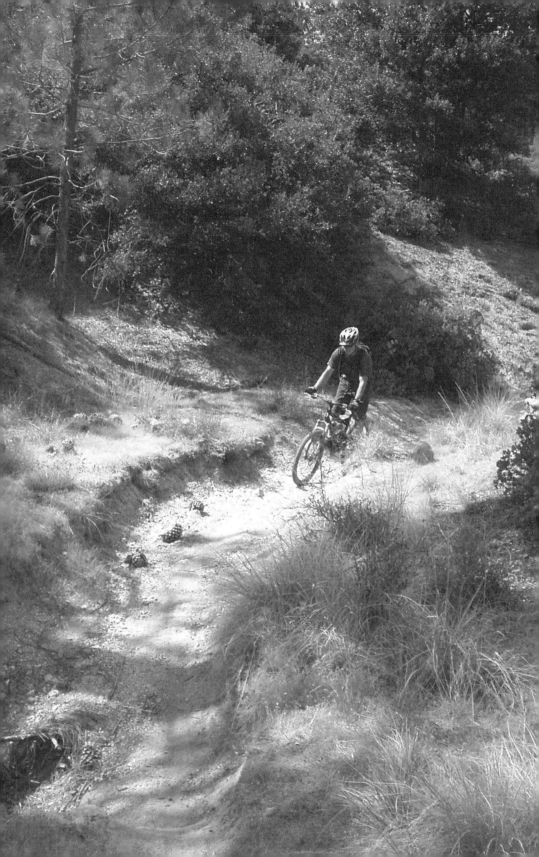

INTRODUCTION

What's Inside

The crux of this book is detailed information on 40 separate mountain bike rides. The chapters of the book represent major riding areas within the county. There may be several trailheads for each riding area and even some individual rides may have multiple trailhead options.

The Overview Map and Overview-map Key

Use the overview map on the inside front cover to assess the location of each ride's primary trailhead. Each ride's number appears on the overview map, on the map key facing the overview map, in the table of contents, and at the top of the ride description's pages.

Trail Maps

Each ride contains a detailed map that shows the trailhead, the route, significant features, facilities, and topographic landmarks such as creeks, overlooks, and peaks. The author gathered map data by carrying a Garmin Etrex Legend C GPS unit while riding. GPS data was downloaded into a digital mapping program—*National Geographic* Topo!—and processed by expert cartographers to produce the highly accurate maps found in this book. Each trailhead's GPS coordinates are included with each profile (see below).

Elevation Profiles

Corresponding directly to the trail map, each ride contains a detailed elevation profile. The elevation profile provides a quick look at the trail from the side, enabling you to visualize how it rises and falls. Note the number of feet between each tick mark on the vertical axis (the height scale). To avoid making flat rides look steep and steep rides appear flat, appropriate height scales are used throughout the book to provide an accurate image of the ride's climbing difficulty. Elevation profiles for loop rides show total distance; those for out-and-back rides show only one-way distance.

GPS Trailhead Coordinates

In addition to GPS-based topographic maps, this book also includes the GPS coordinates for each trailhead in two formats: latitude–longitude and UTM (Universal Transverse Mercator). Latitude–longitude coordinates employ a grid system that indicates your location by means of points along intersecting east–west and north–south lines. Lines of latitude are parallel and run in an east–west direction; the zero-degree line of latitude is the equator.

Lines of longitude are not parallel, run in a north–south direction, and converge at the North and South poles; the zero-degree line of longitude passes through Greenwich, England.

Topographic maps show latitude and longitude as well as UTM grid lines. Known as UTM coordinates, the numbers index a specific point, also using a grid method. The survey information, or datum, used to arrive at the coordinates in this book is WGS84 (versus NAD27 or WGS83). For readers who own a GPS unit, whether handheld or on board a vehicle, the latitude–longitude or UTM coordinates provided on the first page of each ride may be entered into the GPS unit. Just make sure your GPS unit is set to navigate using WGS84 datum. Now you can navigate directly to the trailhead.

Trailheads in parking areas can be reached by car, but some rides still require a short walk or ride to reach the official trailhead from the parking area. In those cases, a handheld unit is necessary to continue the GPS navigation process. That said, readers can easily access all trailheads in this book without a GPS unit by using the directions given, the overview map, and the trail map, which shows at least one significant road leading into the area. But for those who enjoy using the latest GPS technology to navigate, the necessary data have been provided. A brief explanation of the UTM coordinates for El Moro Canyon/Crystal Cove State Park (page 142) follows:

UTM Zone   11S

Easting   423729

Northing   3714404

The UTM zone number **11** refers to one of the 60 vertical zones of the UTM projection, each of which is 6 degrees wide. The UTM zone letter **S** refers to horizontal zones, each of which is 8 degrees wide except for Zone X (12 degrees wide). The easting number **423729** indicates in meters how far east or west a point is from the central meridian of the zone. Increasing easting coordinates on a topographic map or on your GPS screen indicate that you are moving east; decreasing easting coordinates indicate that you are moving west. The northing number **3714404** references in meters how far you are from the equator. Increasing northing coordinates indicate you are traveling north; decreasing northing coordinates indicate you are traveling south. To learn more about how to enhance your outdoor experiences with GPS technology, refer to *GPS Outdoors: A Practical Guide for Outdoor Enthusiasts* (Menasha Ridge Press).

Ride Descriptions

Each ride description contains a detailed description of the route from beginning to end. The ride descriptions are the heart of this book. In each, the author provides a summary of the trail's essence and highlights any extras the ride has to offer. The route is clearly described, including landmarks, side trips, and possible alternate routes along the way. The main narrative is enhanced with an "In Brief" description of the ride, a Key At-a-Glance Information box, and driving directions to the trailhead. Many rides include an "After the Ride" note on nearby activities, such as where to grab a cold brew after the ride.

In Brief

A "taste of the ride"—a snapshot focused on the historic landmarks, scenic vistas, and other sights you may encounter on the trail.

Key At-a-Glance Information

This comprises quick statistics and specifics of each ride:

Length The length of the ride from start to finish (total distance traveled). There may be options to shorten or extend the ride, but the mileage corresponds to the ride as described. Consult the ride description for help deciding on how to customize the ride for your ability or time constraints.

Configuration A description of the layout of the ride. Rides can be loops, out-and-backs, modified loops, or shuttle rides.

Aerobic difficulty The physical effort needed to complete the ride. Rides are generally listed as easy, moderate, difficult, and very difficult. A brief explanation accompanies the rating.

Technical difficulty The riding skill necessary to complete the ride. Rides are rated as easy, moderate, difficult, or extreme. A brief explanation details the nature of the trail's difficulties. Some rides, rated as varied, may have options for riders of different skill levels. Some relatively difficult rides may be suitable for beginners if they are willing to dismount and walk sections that are beyond their abilities. Always ride within your limits and the limits of your bike. There is no shame in walking difficult terrain.

Exposure How much direct sunlight you can expect to encounter during the ride.

Scenery A short summary of what to expect in terms of plant life, wildlife, natural wonders, and scenic vistas

Trail traffic Indicates how busy the ride might be on an average day. Trail traffic, of course, varies from day to day and season to season. Weekend days typically see the most visitors.

Trail surface Indicates whether the trail surface is paved, rocky, gravel, dirt, or a mixture of elements, followed by the percentage of the total route that is singletrack.

Riding time The length of time it takes to complete the ride. The riding time is given as a range. The smaller number is an estimate of how long it would take for a faster rider to complete a route, and the larger number represents how long for a slower rider, for example, "4–6 hours." Usually, the smaller number is the amount of time it took the author to complete the ride. The author is not an extremely fast rider but manages well-above-average speed on both climbs and descents.

Access A notation of any fees or permits that may be needed to access the trail or park at the trailhead.

Maps The name(s) of relevant USGS topo maps and/or maps available at trailheads.

Special comments Any information or tips that are unique to the particular area covered in the profile.

Directions

Used in conjunction with the overview map, the driving directions lead you to the trailhead. Once at the trailhead, park only in designated areas.

After the Ride

An unbiased recommendation of where to eat or drink after riding in a particular area.

Weather

The weather in Los Angeles County and the surrounding areas is mild enough for year-round outdoor recreation. More often than not, heavy precipitation, rather than extreme high or low temperatures, will stop you from riding. Precipitation increases with elevation in Southern California, so always expect more rainfall or snowfall than the local forecasts predict. To be prepared in case of a rainstorm, wear long-sleeved jerseys and long, tight pants for the lower temperatures, and have a light rain jacket in your hydration pack for excessive downpours. Snowfall occurs only about once every decade in the higher elevations of the Santa Monica Mountains, so you'll need to prepare for snowfall only in the higher inland mountains of the Los Padres and Angeles national forests. In those cases, the temperatures will obviously be lower, so prepare accordingly with thicker socks, gloves, and some sort of scarf to protect you from chilling winds. Because Southern California is an arid environment, rainfall will rarely occur between May and November.

The average-temperature chart below refers to temperatures at the Los Angeles Civic Center. For the most part, you can expect lower temps in the higher elevations. However, because they are so close to the great temperature stabilizer that is the Pacific Ocean, in the winter months the Santa Monica Mountains will have higher temperatures than comparable elevations in other mountain ranges described in this book. In the summer months, the opposite can be true. Sometimes the only places with mild temperatures in the dead heat of summer are places close to the ocean. For example, Sycamore and El Moro canyons can be as much as 20 degrees cooler than inland areas on hot days. If you want to beat the heat in the summer, pick a route from this guide that starts within 5 miles of the beach. Remember to slather on the sunblock and bring as much water as you can carry on those really hot days.

Average Temperature by Month (Degrees Fahrenheit)

	January	February	March	April	May	June
High	68.3	67.4	68.8	71.1	73	77.1
Low	48.4	49.7	51.1	53.5	56.5	59.7

	July	August	September	October	November	December
High	82.4	83.2	81.8	77.6	73	67.7
Low	63.1	64	62.7	58.8	53.4	49.4

There really is no mountain biking season in the vicinity of Los Angeles County. It's simply a matter of each rider's preference. Some prefer riding in the heat, and some prefer riding in the cooler temps. Perhaps the best compromise comes in the spring, when the temperatures are mildest and there's still enough moisture in the soil to eliminate sand and dust. Despite SoCal's temperate climate, however, people still die of hypothermia in the Angeles National Forest every once in a while because they weren't prepared to deal with sudden weather changes. Always prepare for the worst in the winter, even going so far as to dress as you would if you were planning on spending the night outside. A hydration pack with prodigious storage space will allow you to carry all the foul-weather gear you need. There's simply no good excuse for not owning one—there are many on the market, and they're affordable.

Water

Always err on the side of excess when deciding how much water to pack: A rider working hard in 90-degree heat needs about ten quarts of fluid per day. That's about 2.5 gallons. In other words, pack one or two bottles, even for short rides. For long rides, especially in hot weather, consider carrying water on your back in a hydration system.

Plan each ride as if there will be zero opportunities to refill your water bottles or hydration packs. Always carry more water than you think you'll need since you never can predict the outcome of your ride. The author has learned through trial and error to carry a full 100-ounce hydration pack with him on every ride exceeding 10 miles in length or with more than 1,500 feet of elevation gain. It is strongly recommended that, when riding any route you're not familiar with, you bring 100 ounces of water because you could get lost, or at the very least make a wrong turn that doubles your aerobic output and need for water. Water bottles, although common, really aren't the way to go. They hold far less water than hydration packs, are tougher to drink from while riding, and can be easily knocked out of their cage and lost on a technical descent. If you can spare the cash, buy a hydration pack with no fewer than 100 ounces of capacity.

Even where water is available, choosing to drink it comes with risks. Some riders are prepared to purify water found along the route. Purifiers with ceramic filters and charcoal prefilters are most efficient at removing bugs and chemicals. You can also pack along the slightly distasteful tetraglycine-hydroperiodide tablets (sold under names such as Potable Aqua and Coughlan's) to debug water.

If you drink found water, the most common waterborne "bug" you'll face is giardia, which may not hit for one to four weeks. Giardia will have you living in the bathroom, passing noxious rotten-egg gas, vomiting, and shivering. Other parasites to worry about include E. coli and cryptosporidium.

For most people, the pleasures of riding make carrying water a relatively minor price to pay to remain healthy. If you're tempted to drink found water, you should do so only if you understand the risks involved. Better yet, hydrate prior to your ride, carry (and drink) eight ounces of water for every mile you ride, and hydrate after the ride.

Clothing

Dressing for mountain biking in Southern California is an enviable experience. For much of the year, the weather is warm and fair, so most days require little more than bike shorts and a short-sleeved jersey. As far as materials are concerned, avoid cotton on all but the hottest days, and never wear cotton socks. Cotton, unlike synthetic or wool fibers, holds moisture. This means that whatever cotton item you are wearing will be soaked with sweat early into your ride and won't dry for the duration. This may not be a problem for the hottest days, but imagine how cold you'll be if the temperature drops or if you get stranded. As a general rule, even on warm days, bring a long-sleeved, cold-weather bike jersey or windbreaker. If they aren't needed to keep you warm, they offer great arm protection on narrow trails with dense foliage and can provide minor protection on long descents, in case of a crash. Rare cold days may require leg warmers or tights, insulated gloves, a long-sleeved insulated jersey, and a lightweight windbreaker.

The Essentials

One of the first rules of riding is to be prepared for anything. The simplest way to be prepared is to carry the essentials. In addition to carrying the items listed on the next page, you need to know how to use them, especially the navigation items. Always consider worst-case scenarios such as getting lost, riding back in the dark, breaking components, cracking a wrist, or encountering a brutal thunderstorm. The items listed below don't cost a lot of money, don't take up much room in a pack, and don't weigh much—but they might just save your life.

- **Compass** (and a GPS unit if you have one)
- **Extra clothes:** rain protection, warm layers, gloves, and a warm hat
- **Extra food:** you should always have some left when you've finished riding
- **Fire:** windproof matches or a lighter and fire starter
- **First-aid kit:** a compact, good-quality kit including first-aid instructions
- **Knife:** a bike multitool with a knife is best
- **Light:** flashlight or headlamp, with extra bulbs and batteries
- **Map:** preferably a topo map and a copy of this book's trail maps and ride descriptions
- **Mirror:** to attract attention from aircraft in emergencies
- **Sun protection:** sunglasses, lip balm, sunblock, and a sun hat (in case you have to walk)
- **Water:** durable bottles and water treatment such as iodine or a filter

Topo Maps

The maps in this book have been produced with great care and, used with the hiking directions, will direct you to the trail and help you stay on course. However, you will find additional detail and valuable information in the United States Geological Survey's 7.5-minute series topographic maps. Topo maps are available online in many locations. The downside to USGS topos is that many of them are outdated, having been created 20 to 30 years ago. Cultural features on outdated topo maps, such as roads, will probably be inaccurate, but the topographic features should be accurate.

Digital topographic-map programs such as DeLorme's TopoUSA enable you to review topo maps of the entire United States on your PC. Gathered while hiking with a tracking unit, GPS data can be downloaded using the software, allowing you to plot your own hikes. Google Earth (**earth.google.com**) is a great free program that lets you check aerial views against a topo map.

If you're new to maps, you might be wondering what a topo map is. In short, it indicates not only linear distance but elevation as well, using contour lines. Each squiggly brown line represents a particular elevation, and at the base of each topo, a contour's interval designation is given. If the contour interval is 20 feet, then the distance between each contour line is 20 feet. Follow five contour lines up on the same map, and the elevation has increased by 100 feet. Every fifth contour line is labeled with an altitude. These lines are slightly heavier than the intervening contour lines and are called the index lines. An index line that reads "1,300" indicates a contour that is 1,300 feet above sea level.

In addition to the outdoor shops listed in the Appendix, sources for topos include major universities and some public libraries, where you can photocopy the maps you need to avoid the cost of buying them. But if you want your own and can't find them locally, visit the United States Geological Survey's Web site, **topomaps.usgs.gov.**

Bike Tools

Even for short rides, carrying these basics requires only a small seat bag or stem bag. The most common problem is probably the dreaded flat. If you opt for carrying only compressed air to reinflate tires, you run the risk of having more flats than you have air cylinders. A small collapsible pump solves that problem. Before you go, make sure your tire-patch kit's rubber cement hasn't dried out. Planning for three flats on every ride isn't excessive because there are many small, thorn-producing shrubs in SoCal. Plus, you can't always count on your riding buddies or strangers on the trail to be so adequately prepared. If your chain snaps, you'll need a chain tool, extra pins, and possibly a small length of new chain to piece it back together.

- Chain tool
- Duct tape
- Multitool
- Patch kit
- Spare tube
- Tire pump and/or compressed-air kit with no fewer than three air cartridges
- Tire lever
- Zip ties

The multitool should address the balance of repairs or adjustments (seat, brakes, and/or derailleurs) you may need to make on a ride. If you snap your frame in half, just call it a day and don't bother with the tools.

First-aid Kit

A very basic first-aid kit may contain more items than you might think necessary. Prepackaged kits in waterproof bags are available (Atwater Carey and Adventure Medical make a variety of kits). Though there are quite a few items listed here, they pack into a small space:

- Ace bandages for sprains or to make compression bandages
- Antibiotic ointment (Neosporin or the generic equivalent) for cuts
- Aspirin or acetaminophen for aches
- Band-Aids for cuts
- Benadryl or the generic equivalent, diphenhydramine (in case of allergic reactions)
- Butterfly-closure bandages for deep cuts
- Epinephrine in a prefilled syringe (for people known to have severe allergic reactions to such things as bee stings)
- Roll of gauze to secure bandages
- Gauze compress pads (a half dozen 4 x 4–inch pads) to clean and cover wounds
- Hydrogen peroxide or iodine for cuts and abrasions
- Insect repellent, in case the bugs are on holiday with you
- Matches or a pocket lighter to build fires for warmth or to heat water or cook food
- Sunscreen to prevent sunburn
- Whistle (it's more effective in signaling rescuers than your voice is)

General Safety

Potentially dangerous situations can occur, but preparation and sound judgment make for safer forays into remote and wild areas. Here are a few tips.

- Make sure your car, truck, or SUV is in good shape before you go to the park, and check road conditions before you set out. If your vehicle breaks down, stay with it—it's easier to find a vehicle than a person.
- Always carry food and water, whether you are planning an overnight trip or not. Food will give you energy, help keep you warm, and sustain you in an emergency situation until help arrives. Always bring water, or boil, filter, or treat found water before drinking it.
- Wear sturdy biking shoes.
- Wear a professional-grade bike helmet (brain bucket).

- Never ride alone—take a buddy with you on the trails.
- Tell someone where you're going and when you'll be back (be as specific as possible), and ask him or her to get help if you don't return in a reasonable amount of time.
- Stay on the trails and routes described in this book. Most riders get lost when they leave the path. Even on the most clearly marked trails, there is usually a point where you have to stop and consider which direction to head. If you become disoriented, don't panic. As soon as you think you may be off track, stop, assess your current direction, and then retrace your path to the point where you went astray. Using a map, a compass, and this book, and keeping in mind what you have already passed, reorient yourself and trust your judgment on which way to continue. If you become absolutely unsure of how to proceed, return to your vehicle the way you came. Should you become completely lost and have no idea of how to return to the trailhead, remaining in place along the trail and waiting for help is most often the best choice for adults and always the best option for kids. If you have prepared well, brought supplies, and taken that all-important step of telling someone where you'll be and for how long, staying in place shouldn't result in disaster.
- Take along your brain. A cool, calculating mind is the single most important piece of equipment you'll need on the trail. Think before you act. Watch your step. Plan ahead. Avoiding accidents altogether is the best recipe for a rewarding and relaxing ride.
- Ask questions. It's a lot easier to get advice beforehand and avoid mishaps away from civilization, where finding help may be difficult.

Ticks

Although tick-borne Lyme disease is not nearly as common in California as in the northeastern United States, several cases are reported here each year, according to the U.S. Centers for Disease Control and Prevention (CDC). Although extremely low in California, the risk is enough to make postride tick checks mandatory. Ticks, commonly found in brushy and woodsy areas, are arthropods, not insects, and they need a host in order to reproduce. The ticks that light onto you while you ride will be very small—sometimes so tiny that you won't be able to spot them. Primarily of two varieties, deer ticks and dog ticks, they need a few hours of actual attachment before they can transmit any disease. Ticks may settle in shoes, socks, or hats. The best strategy is to visually check every so often while riding, do a thorough check before you get in the car, and then, when you take a postride shower, do an even more thorough check of your entire body. Ticks that haven't attached are easily removed but not easily killed. If you pick off a tick while on the trail, just toss it aside. If you find one on your body at home, remove it and then send it down the toilet. For ticks that have become embedded, removal with tweezers is best.

Snakes

Of the many snakes that inhabit the mountains and foothills of Southern California, the only species that is of any danger to humans is the rattlesnake. It is a common and dangerous misconception that rattlesnakes will rattle when encountered or provoked. Increasingly frequent are accounts of the common Southern Pacific rattlesnake's remaining silent even when surrounded. To avoid being bitten, simply don't mess with any snake. When you see one crossing a trail, just stop and allow it to get out of the way. Snakes are probably the most common wildlife encountered, so enjoy and respect them. On warm days in the Santa Monica Mountains, it's possible to see several rattlers in one day without looking hard. Be wary of rattlesnakes when entering any area that would be a good hiding place for them—under rocks, under foliage, and in grassy areas.

Mountain Lions

If you live in Southern California, you probably remember the mountain lion attacks of 2004 at Whiting Ranch Wilderness Park in Orange County, in which one rider was killed and another injured. The culprit turned out to be a 120-pound male mountain lion—proven to be the killer when human remains were found in its stomach after it was hunted down. This sobering story does not reflect the true rarity of mountain lion attacks, much less encounters. Between 1890 and 2004, there were only 16 attacks and 7 fatalities recorded in the state of California, according to Wikipedia.org. However, virtually all the routes described in this book are in mountain lion territory. Either accept that fact and enjoy mountain biking, or stay at home and play video games.

Here are a few helpful guidelines for handling potential mountain lion encounters:

- Keep kids close to you. Observed in captivity, mountain lions seem especially drawn to small children.
- Do not run from a mountain lion. Running may stimulate the animal's instinct to chase.
- Don't approach a mountain lion—give him room to get away.
- Try to make yourself look larger by raising your arms and/or opening your jacket if you're wearing one.
- Do not crouch or kneel. These movements could make you look smaller and more like the mountain lion's prey.
- Try to convince the mountain lion you are dangerous—not its prey. Without crouching, gather nearby stones or branches and toss them at the animal. Slowly wave your arms above your head and speak in a firm voice.
- If all fails and you are attacked, fight back. People have successfully fought off attacking mountain lions with rocks and sticks. Try to remain facing the animal, and fend off its attempts to bite your head or neck—the lion's typical aim.

Poison Oak

Poison oak is primarily recognizable by its three-leaflet configuration—on either a vine or shrub. However, during the fall and winter months, poison oak can be more elusive because the telltale leaves fall off, and little more than a stem protrudes from the ground. This is why the worst rash afflictions occur in the cooler months. Usually within 12 to 14 hours of exposure (but sometimes much later), raised lines and/or blisters will appear, accompanied by a terrible itch. Urushiol, the oil in the sap of this plant, is responsible for the rash. Refrain from scratching, since bacteria under fingernails can cause infection; you can also spread the rash to other parts of your body by scratching. Wash and dry the rash thoroughly, applying a calamine lotion or other product to help dry it. If the itching or blistering is severe, seek medical attention. Remember that oil-contaminated clothes, pets, or riding gear can easily cause an irritating rash on you or someone else, so be sure to wash exposed parts of your body and exposed clothing, gear, and pets.

Trail Etiquette

Whether you're on a city, county, state, or national park trail, always remember that great care and resources (from nature as well as from your tax dollars) have gone into creating these trails. Treat the trail, wildlife, and your fellow riders with respect.

- Ride on open trails only. Respect trail and road closures (ask if you're not sure), avoid trespassing on private land, obtain permits and authorization as required, and leave gates as you found them or as marked.
- Leave only tire prints. Pack out what you pack in. No one likes to see the trash someone else has left behind.
- Never intentionally spook animals. An unannounced approach, a sudden movement, or a loud noise startles most animals. A surprised animal can be dangerous to you, others, and the animal itself.
- Plan ahead. Know your bike, your ability, and the area in which you are riding—and prepare accordingly. Be self-sufficient at all times; carry necessary supplies for changes in weather or other conditions.
- Be courteous to other riders, equestrians, and all others you encounter on the trails; maintaining a wide grin makes this task a lot easier.

Mountain Bike Technology

Originally, mountain bikes were simply road bikes adapted for off-road use. They retained the same cable-pull brake systems as road bikes and lacked suspension of any kind. Cut to the modern day, in which a typical cross-country mountain bike has 4 to 6 inches of suspension travel on both ends and is equipped with hydraulic disc brakes. These innovations are anything but gimmicky technology. Disc brakes and suspension will undoubtedly enhance your riding experiences. There are, however, some crucial adjustments and maintenance involved that mountain bikers and shops alike often overlook.

Setting Up Your Suspension

Mountain bike suspension technology is very similar to what's found on modern motocross and off-road motorcycles. In fact, the technology was directly borrowed from the motorcycle industry. Knowing this, it's astonishing how few mountain bikers set up their suspension correctly for their weight. All serious motocross riders and amateur, professional, or weekend warriors have their bikes sprung properly for their weight before taking a single lap on the track. Mountain bikers must do the same, or their bikes will not handle properly. Suspension, when correctly sprung, is supposed to inspire confidence, enhance control, and ensure comfort. Incorrectly sprung suspension will not. Suspension setup is simple and crucial.

If your bike is air sprung, just borrow a shock pump from someone and set your bike's fork and rear shock to the appropriate PSI for your weight, according to the manufacturer's specifications. Since rear-shock setup varies with frame design, contact the frame manufacturer for information. For setting up forks, just contact the manufacturer directly.

Setting up a bike with coil-sprung forks and rear shocks is a little more difficult but still no big deal. Virtually every coil-sprung suspension system comes with springs that are only stiff enough for riders around the 160-pound mark. Since the window is very small, a 130-pound rider will find the ride stiff and unforgiving, while a 200-pound rider will feel the bike sag to the depths of its travel and bottom out over the smallest bumps and drops. If this problem isn't addressed, neither the lighter nor the heavier rider will be able to enjoy the benefits of the suspension systems he or she paid big bucks for. If your weight is outside the "window," simply order stiffer springs from the manufacturer and have the bike shop install them, or do it yourself. Problem solved.

Damping systems are the other crucial component of suspension systems. Fortunately, they are not weight-specific. The amount of adjustability typically increases with cost. The most common knob found on rear shocks and forks is the "rebound" adjuster. Turning the knob in one direction will slow the speed at which the shock or fork returns to full extension after being compressed by the rider or hitting a bump. Turn the knob in the other direction and the shock or fork will extend more quickly. In most cases, you should turn the knob the correct number of turns so it is in the middle—not slowest or fastest—and make minute adjustments from there. If you favor downhilling and want your suspension to react to every bump, you'll generally want faster rebound damping. If you don't want your suspension bobbing or bouncing as you pedal, slower rebound will help. Rarely will you ride with the rebound adjusted to the slowest or fastest speed. Too-slow rebound will not allow the shock to react to consecutive bumps—after the first impact, the shock will not extend enough to absorb the second impact. Not enough rebound damping will make the bike squirrelly and too vulnerable to braking and pedaling inputs.

Some of the more expensive and fancier shocks and forks allow for adjustment of "compression" damping. Simply put, adjusting the "compression" dictates how fast the shock or fork will compress into its stroke. As with rebound, climbers will generally want slower compression for efficiency, and downhillers will opt for faster compression for better bump absorption. Compression that is set too fast will cause the suspension to compress too fast, while slow compression will make the suspension too harsh and nonreactive. Setting up compression is just like setting up rebound; just start in the middle range and make small adjustments to suit your needs.

Once set up properly, suspension forks and shocks typically have a very long operational lifespan. Eventually, perhaps after 1,000 miles of heavy use, you should change the oil. The seals should also be inspected and/or changed at this juncture. Oil leaks are rare, but they do occur and are most often the result of expired seals. Don't worry; seals are cheap and easy to get. Trust me—changing seals and suspension oil is a messy job—support your local bike shop and have them do it.

Disc Brakes

When disc brakes were first introduced, many experienced bikers scoffed at the concept. Now many of them are believers, because disc brakes are more reliable and provide better modulation and stopping power than their rim-squeezing predecessors. They also enhance rider safety because they require less effort to use, alleviating the cramping that can build up in fingers on long descents. There is simply no reason to avoid them.

Overall, disc brakes require less maintenance than cable-pull rim brakes do. Once they are set up, you can basically forget about them until it's time to change the pads. Brake pads vary in composition from manufacturer to manufacturer; therefore, they will wear at different rates. To avoid mishap, just check them frequently. Most often, the pads will be visible without your having to remove the wheel. If not, remove the wheel and peer inside the caliper to see how much pad material is left. Make sure you know how much should be there by taking note of how much pad material is present on a new pad.

Despite their benefits, there are two major problems that can occur following improper maintenance of bicycle disc brakes. The most maddening is excessive drag or the hissing sound heard when the brakes aren't applied. This most commonly occurs when a hydraulic caliper is accidentally "pumped out." This almost always happens when the wheel is removed. To avoid this, don't allow your brake lever to be depressed when you're changing a tire. If shipping or transporting the bike over long distances, place something of the same width as the rotor or larger inside the caliper. Hayes, a brake manufacturer, makes a small card-like device for this purpose. Otherwise, several business cards or old credit cards will do. If your pads do accidentally get "pumped out," you will need to push the calipers back to their starting position so they can accommodate the rotor with no drag or squealing. Each manufacturer has a specific, albeit simple, procedure to follow regarding this minor dilemma, so see your user's manuals, check the manufacturer's Web site, or call tech support.

The other major problem caused by improper disc-brake maintenance results from failure to "break in" the new pads before usage. New, unused brake pads will have hardly any stopping power at first. Obviously, this can present a serious danger to the rider. Before you encounter any unpredictable terrain, ride your bike down a long, easy, safe descent while applying moderate brake pressure the whole way. As the pads rub the rotors, they will lose their high spots and flatten, vastly enhancing their stopping power. Pad brake-in may seem like a nuisance, but, remember, this is the same procedure you follow after an automobile brake service. Mechanics don't tell you to "go easy on the brakes for 250 miles" to be annoying: they are trying to save your life. Fortunately, bicycle disc-brake pads can be broken in much more quickly. One half-mile descent will usually get the job done.

In addition to occasional pad changes, owners of bicycle disc-brake systems are also required to "bleed" out the old, used oil of their hydraulic brake systems and replace it with new oil. Fortunately, this messy procedure is necessary only after many thousands of miles of use. Many riders will never bleed their brakes and will nevertheless experience zero problems. As with changing suspension oil, have your local bike shop bleed your brakes to save you the hassle. Users of mechanical, or cable-pull, disc brakes will need to change their cables and cable housing every once in a while, about as often as they change their derailleur cables and housing.

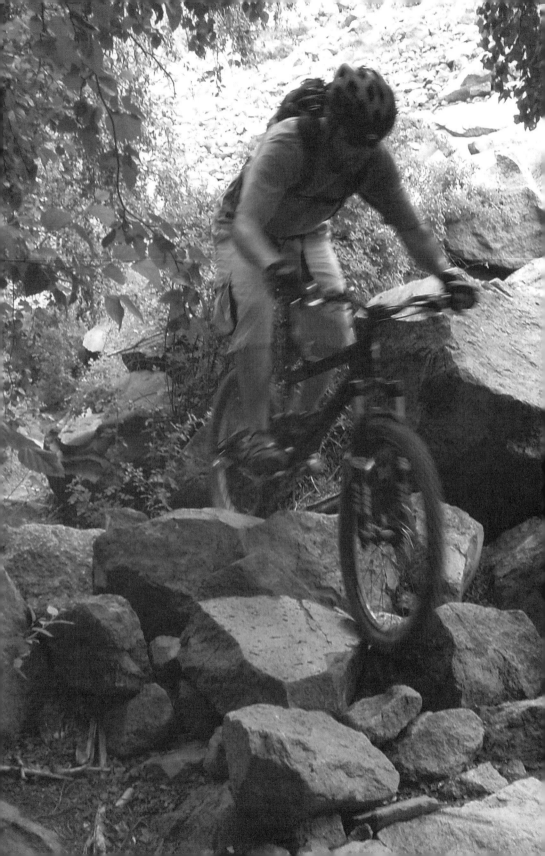

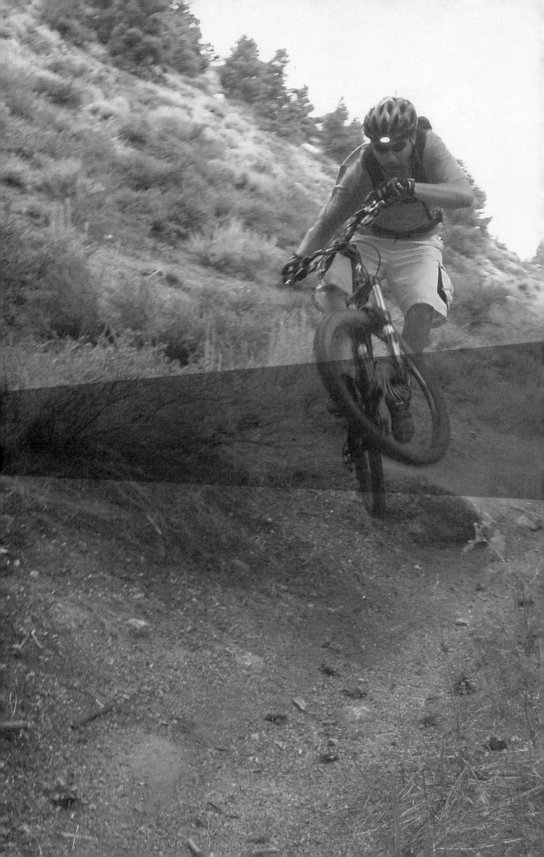

SANTA MONICA MOUNTAINS WEST

KEY AT-A-GLANCE INFORMATION

Length: 16 miles

Configuration: Figure-8

Aerobic difficulty: 4

Technical difficulty: 3

Scenery: Broad views of Oxnard, Sandstone Peak, Point Mugu, Pacific Ocean

Exposure: Fully exposed to sunshine for 80% of ride, some shade in lower areas of Big Sycamore Canyon Fire Road

Trail traffic: Moderate during weekdays, heavy on weekends

Trail surface: Approximately 30% singletrack, 70% fire road; mostly hard-packed and dry

Riding time: 2–3 hours

Access: Sunrise–sunset, 7 days a week

Maps: USGS 7.5-minute quads: Camarillo, Point Mugu

Special comments: Parking fee is $10. Ample free parking can be found along Pacific Coast Highway north and south of the area.

GPS TRAILHEAD COORDINATES (WGS84)
UTM Zone   11S
Easting   314150
Northing   3772292
Latitude   N 34.04'30"
Longitude   W 119.00'51"

BIG SYCAMORE CANYON

In Brief

Big Sycamore Canyon, located in the northernmost region of the Santa Monica Mountains in the Point Mugu State Park, contains a variety of trails well suited to riders of all skill levels. The pristine, quintessential California beach at the mouth of Big Sycamore Creek is a great distraction for nonriders coming along for the day. Big Sycamore Canyon, in addition to being a great place to bring the whole family, stays drastically cooler than the rest of LA County's rides on hot summer days. After you experience the Guadalasca and Backbone trails, arguably the most entertaining singletrack in the Santa Monica Mountains, you may not want to go home at the end of the day, and you don't have to because there are several great campsites.

Description

Once inside the campsite, follow the signs to the trailhead, which starts at the northern end of the campgrounds, roughly one-quarter mile from the Pacific Coast Highway (PCH). Big Sycamore Canyon Trail is a wide, flat fire road with heavy bicycle, hiker, and equestrian traffic, so take it easy here. Spin your way to the entrance to the Overlook Trail, which will be on your left side, about 0.4 miles from the entrance to Big Sycamore.

Clean ocean air, pleasant views of the Pacific Ocean, and unmolested chaparral make the Overlook Trail one of

DIRECTIONS

The best way to access this ride is to stage from the Sycamore Canyon Campground, located 15 miles south of Oxnard on CA 1 (Pacific Coast Highway) or, if coming from Los Angeles, 32.2 miles north of where Interstate 10 Freeway terminates to CA 1 in Santa Monica.

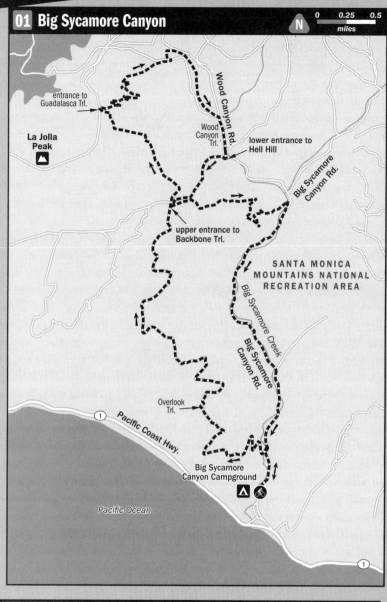

0   0.25   0.5
miles

N

La Jolla Peak

entrance to Guadalasca Trl.

Wood Canyon Rd.

Wood Canyon Trl.

lower entrance to Hell Hill

Big Sycamore Canyon Rd.

upper entrance to Backbone Trl.

SANTA MONICA MOUNTAINS NATIONAL RECREATION AREA

Big Sycamore Creek

Big Sycamore Canyon Rd.

Overlook Trl.

Pacific Coast Hwy.

1

Big Sycamore Canyon Campground

Pacific Ocean

1

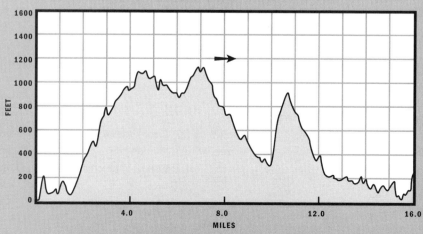

the sweetest ascents to be found anywhere in SoCal. The climbing is tough, but not relentless because a few flat spots will alleviate the pain in your lungs and legs along the way. Sandstone Peak dominates the skyline to the east, rising to 3,117 feet, making it the highest mountain in the Santa Monica Mountain range.

If you've had enough after 4.5 miles of the Overlook Trail, you have two bailout options. You can either descend the Backbone Trail, which will be clearly marked with a sign on your right, or go down Hell Hill, which is a fire road, also on the right about 300 feet beyond Backbone. Hell Hill is a steep beeline back to Big Sycamore, and much easier than the twisty, bumpy singletrack that is Backbone. If you have the grit, avoid bailing out here and continue up Overlook for another 1.25 miles so you can be rewarded with the Guadalasca singletrack descent. The views become more and more interesting near the summit of Overlook, at the top of which you can survey the vast agricultural plains of Oxnard.

After a brief downhill, look for the entrance to Guadalasca Trail on your right at the end of Overlook. Guadalasca is crazy fun and a great training ground for the more advanced, technical singletrack descents you will find in other less-forgiving areas of LA County, such as the San Gabriel Mountains. Watch for tight switchbacks you can crash on—without falling off a cliff—and don't hesitate to turn around and give them another run if you dab or fall. The dense vegetation can obscure your view, so resist flying at warp speed because many riders choose this trail as their ascent. Unfortunately, this utopian section ends after roughly 2.5 miles at Wood Canyon Trail, where you turn right.

Savor the next 0.3-mile-long section of Wood Canyon Trail to the fullest because when you turn right and ascend the infamous Hell Hill Fire Road, you'll beg for mercy and dream of the next descent. Aptly named, Hell Hill gains roughly 650 feet in 0.7 miles. If you're on a single-speed bike, this will be a hiking section for you or anyone else who left their granny gear at home. Climbing this hill without dabbing is a true accomplishment and will give you a pass to climb any hill in Southern California—it just doesn't get tougher than this. If you're still pedaling at the halfway mark, you will be rewarded with a whopper endorphin rush that may have you calling it "Heaven Hill" from that point forward. If you somehow pedaled to the top on a mono-cogger, please contact Menasha Ridge Press for a free T-shirt and trail guide ($50 shipping). Better yet, look in the mirror to make sure you're not Ned Overend.

After rewarding yourself with a snack and gloating about your accomplishment to your buddies and crowning yourself king of the Santa Monica mountain range, hang a left onto Overlook Trail and make another left so you can take your victory lap down the Backbone Trail. This section of the Backbone is a hoot, with less speed-limiting foliage than the Guadalasca Trail. Smooth-banked turns rather than tight switchbacks make this chute reminiscent of a toboggan run. Play it safe, though; this is not the Winter Olympics, and you'll need to watch for plenty of uphill traffic. After about 1.7 miles, cross Big Sycamore Creek and rejoin the Big Sycamore Canyon Trail.

The last 3 miles of your ride rattle down the Big Sycamore Canyon Trail, which is wide, groomed, and subdued. Several creek crossings, however, will keep you vigilant in the spring and winter when water is present. You return to your point of origin about 14.5

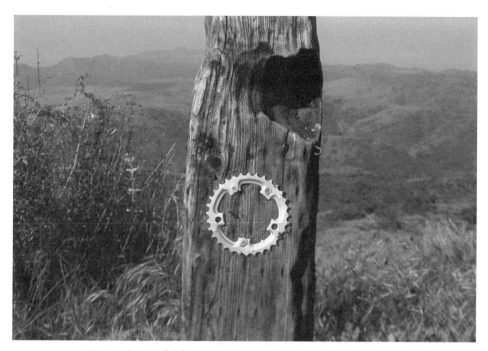

Some nice trailside artwork near the summit at Sycamore

laughter-, sweat-, blood-, and tear-drenched miles later, and reward yourself with the cold beverage you so deftly placed in the cooler at your staging area.

After the Ride

Big Sycamore Canyon Trail is pretty remote, so your best bet is to treat yourself to a portable feast. If you didn't adequately prepare, travel 3.2 miles south to Neptune's Net Seafood at 42505 Pacific Coast Highway for a fatty spread of fried seafood and frosty brews; (310) 457-3095. This classic landmark, just across from the famous LA County–line surf spot, is filled with bikers and tourists on the weekend, so be prepared for a long line to place your order.

O2

EDISON ROAD/ZUMA RIDGE/ BACKBONE TRAIL

KEY AT-A-GLANCE INFORMATION

Length: 11.2 miles

Configuration: Loop

Technical difficulty: 3

Aerobic difficulty: 5

Scenery: Zuma Canyon, Santa Monica Mountains, Zuma Ridge, Trancas Canyon

Exposure: 80% exposed to sunshine

Trail traffic: Virtually nonexistent on Edison Road and Zuma Ridge, moderate on Backbone Trail

Trail surface: Dry hardpack with some loose, rocky sections— 20% singletrack

Riding time: 2.5–3.5 hours

Access: Sunrise–sunset, 7 days a week

Maps: USGS 7.5-minute quad: Point Dume

Special comments: Don't embark on this ride if you're a novice— once you get to Zuma Creek, you must make 2 very tough climbs to get out.

GPS TRAILHEAD COORDINATES (WGS84)

UTM Zone   11S
Easting   333526
Northing   377444
Latitude   N 34.03'41"
Longitude   W 118.48'14"

In Brief

It's baffling that so few people ride Edison Road to Zuma Ridge. Perhaps the reason is that the trailhead is concealed on the side of Kanan Dume Road and closed with a fence that, ironically, has a sign welcoming users. Lift your bike over the fence and do this route, because it is one of the wildest, most aerobically challenging rides in the Santa Monica Mountains. Its lack of trail traffic and remote location ensure you a good chance of seeing rare wildlife such as bobcats and horned toads.

Description

Once you've found the elusive entrance to Edison Road, get your gear together and start pedaling. You're in for a small bit of climbing in the first mile, and then at the 1.3-mile mark you'll begin the descent into the depths of Zuma Canyon, during which you'll lose more than 800 feet of elevation. The Edison Fire Road gets an occasional grooming, but it can be pretty rocky and technical for a fire road.

When you cross Zuma Creek at the 3-mile mark, stop and appreciate the wildness of the environment around you—here is an entire canyon that has somehow remained free of urban encroachment despite being situated in the heart of Malibu. Don't stop too long, however; it would behoove you to keep your legs somewhat warm for the monstrous climb ahead—approximately 1,700 feet of elevation to gain over the next 3 miles. If you're

DIRECTIONS

From Los Angeles, take CA 1 (Pacific Coast Highway) north until you reach Kanan Dume Road, then turn right and look out for the entrance to Edison Road, which will appear on your left after about 3 miles. If you have trouble seeing it, follow the power lines on the hillside down to Kanan Dume Road. There is ample parking on the shoulder.

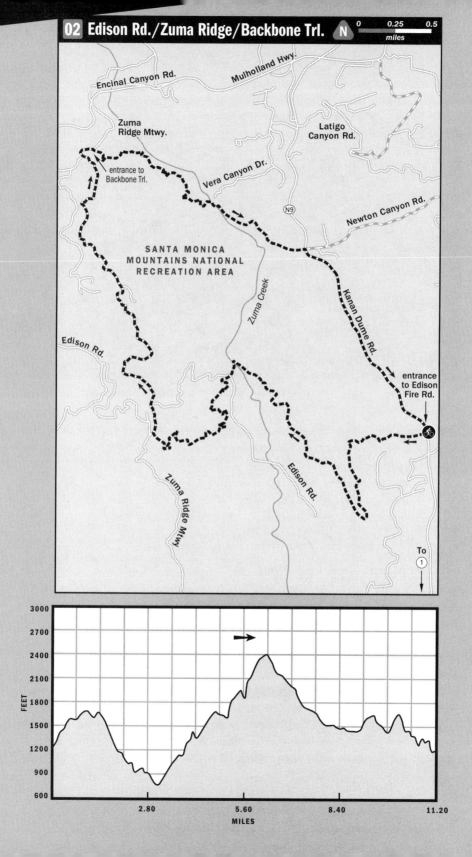

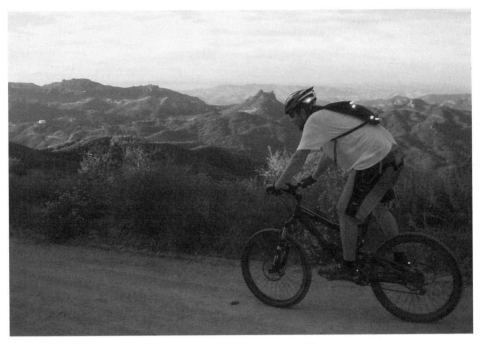

Splendid views aplenty along Zuma Ridge Motorway

in good enough shape to ignore the pain of this climb, you may treat your eyes to a visual feast—about halfway into the climb, the scenery opens up, with Trancas Canyon and the Pacific coming into view.

The lone home at the top marks the summit, after which you descend along Zuma Ridge. The views are spectacular here also, and the fire road is smooth, with fast-sweeping corners to get sideways on. Keep an eye out for the entrance to the Backbone Trail; it will appear on your right at roughly the 7.6-mile mark, about 1.2 miles from the estate atop Zuma Ridge.

The ensuing 2.4 miles of Backbone Trail are a delight, taking you across the upper part of Zuma Creek, then paralleling Kanan Dume Road for a while. This section is quintessential chaparral singletrack, with dead oak leaves contributing to a nice loamy trail surface that provides plenty of grip. This section is particularly popular with hikers, so avoid recklessly high speeds around the numerous blind corners.

Your last mile on the Backbone Trail will leave you euphoric after its nice little oak-canopy-shaded ascent and subsequent descent. Tires will say goodbye to dirt at the 10-mile mark when the last leg of the journey begins—a 1.3-mile southward spin on Kanan Dume Road south back to your car. Mostly downhill, this pavement portage includes two tunnels to keep things interesting. Unless your bike racks drew other cyclists' attention, your car will most likely be as alone as you left it. Edison Road gets very little cycling attention, and when you're done, you'll agree it's deserving of far more.

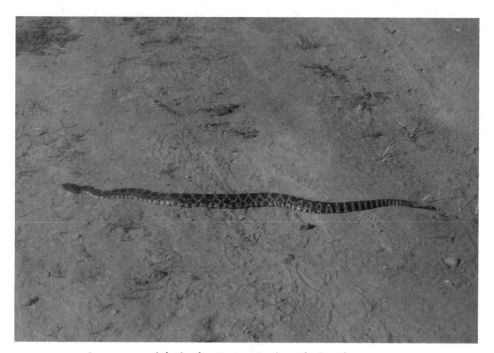

A common sight in the Santa Monicas during the summer

After the Ride

Virtually every international flavor of cuisine can be found on PCH as you head back to Los Angeles. Cholada Thai Beach Cuisine at 18763 Pacific Coast Highway offers fiery fare as well as cold bottled Thai macrobrews to wash it down; (310) 317-0025. For American food, a full bar, and possibly a musical display from forgotten bands of the '80s, visit The Malibu Inn, across from the historical Malibu Pier at 22969 Pacific Coast Highway; (310) 456-6060.

BACKBONE TRAIL: CORRAL CANYON TO KANAN DUME

KEY AT-A-GLANCE INFORMATION

Length: 12.2 Miles

Configuration: Out-and-back

Aerobic difficulty: 4

Technical difficulty: 4

Scenery: Pacific Ocean, Santa Monica Mountains, Castro Peak

Exposure: 80% sunny, shady in creek area

Trail traffic: Light–moderate on weekdays, moderate on weekends

Trail surface: 100% singletrack; varies from loose and dry to hard-packed and loamy

Riding time: 2–3 hours

Access: Sunrise–sunset, 7 days a week

Maps: USGS 7.5-minute quad: Point Dume

Special comments: It can be very hot on this ride, so bring plenty of water and use sunblock.

In Brief

Thanks to advocacy groups like the Concerned Off-Road Bicyclists Association and the International Mountain Bicycling Association, the Backbone Trail is still open to mountain bikers. This section of Backbone is cherished by many as the best singletrack action in the Santa Monica Mountains. If you had only one day to ride in Los Angeles, this would be the place to go. This section of Backbone has everything—challenging climbs, tricky switchbacks, technical creek crossings and shaded, loamy stretches that look as if they were taken right out of your favorite mountain bike magazine.

Description

Although there are a variety of staging options for this ride, the Corral Canyon entrance provides a gradual climb as a warm-up, rather than the very laborious grind (from the Kanan Dume Road entrance at the other end of this route) that will turn your cold legs into Jell-O. Staging from Corral Canyon also saves the most fun for the descent at the end of the ride, which is a theme of the recommended routes in this book.

Two trails are accessible from the Corral Canyon parking lot. One is a fire road called Castro Crest Motorway that leads to Castro Peak. Although at one time this was a scenic option that could be incorporated into the Backbone experience, the connecting fire road called Newton Motorway has since been gated off by the owner

GPS TRAILHEAD COORDINATES (WGS84)

UTM Zone 11S
Easting 337742
Northing 3772637
Latitude N 34.05'55"
Longitude W 118.45'31"

DIRECTIONS

From CA 1 (Pacific Coast Highway), take Corral Canyon Road for 5.4 miles until it terminates in a parking lot. The trailhead is in the southwest end of the small parking lot.

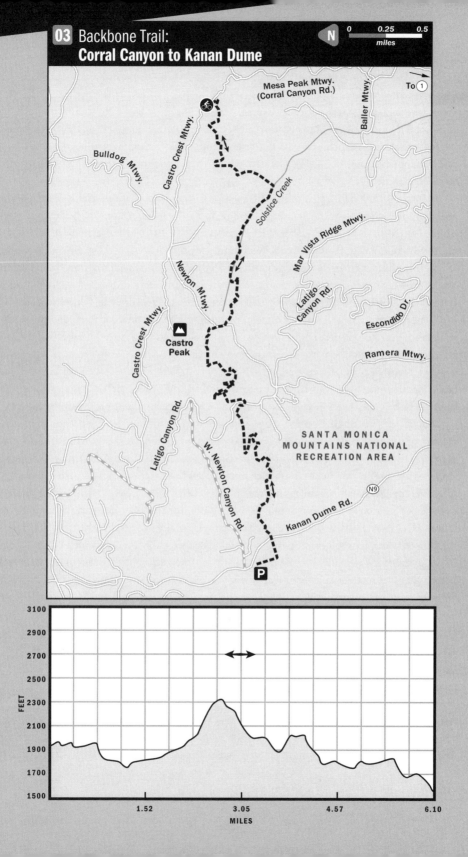

N

0   0.25   0.5
miles

Mesa Peak Mtwy.
(Corral Canyon Rd.)

To (1)

Baller Mtwy.

Castro Crest Mtwy.

Bulldog Mtwy.

Solstice Creek

Mar Vista Ridge Mtwy.

Newton Mtwy.

Latigo
Canyon Rd.

Escondido Dr.

Castro
Peak

Ramera Mtwy.

Castro Crest Mtwy.

Latigo Canyon Rd.

W. Newton Canyon Rd.

SANTA MONICA
MOUNTAINS NATIONAL
RECREATION AREA

(N9)

Kanan Dume Rd.

P

FEET

3100
2900
2700
2500
2300
2100
1900
1700
1500

1.52   3.05   4.57   6.10
MILES

of the radio-tower facility and private residence at the summit. If you ride up this hill, you won't be able to reconnect with Backbone. Fortunately, land disputes have so far spared the Backbone Trail. Its entrance is clearly marked in the western end of the parking area.

The Backbone starts with an easy descent, followed by some light climbing and flat sections. This recently scorched section, although certified singletrack, doesn't do justice to the rest of the ride, which just gets better and better. After about 0.7 miles, you'll descend into the upper reaches of Solstice Canyon, where you'll encounter a few moderately difficult creek crossings.

After your last dab-free crossing of Solstice Creek, shift into the granny gear and get ready for the longest sustained climb of the day. You will ascend nearly 500 feet over the next 0.75 miles, so pace yourself and ponder the meaning of life while you pedal this grinder, gracefully conquering its moderately challenging switchbacks.

At roughly 2.5 miles from your car, cross Newton Motorway and rejoin the Backbone Trail. The next quarter mile has minimal elevation change, but only adept technical riders can ride it dab-free because of some rocky areas with hidden lines of *Da Vinci Code* stature. The next order of business is a steep, winding half-mile descent that you will enjoy a lot more if you don't think about how painful it will be to climb up the other side. At the bottom of this section, cross a creek and see an old, rusty motor scooter made some time ago by a Spanish company called Derbi. If you're completely pooped at this point and have fantasies about ditching your rig and motoring out on this European bad boy, don't bother— the scooter has long since ceased running and now serves as a landmark on this trail.

Cross another staging option when you ride into a parking lot about 4 miles in, after which you'll cross Latigo Canyon Road and continue riding the Backbone. After another grin-inspiring half-mile descent, you'll encounter a rare treat in Southern California—a 0.9-mile stretch with several small climbs and descents, rather than an extreme example of one or the other. At approximately 5.7 miles in, cross a paved private road and 0.2 miles later descend a very steep section of trail into Santa Monica Mountains Conservancy parking lot at Kanan Dume Road. You'll turn around and start backtracking here, but don't take your siesta yet— you'll need warm legs to grind up that horrendously steep hill you just floated down.

Out-and-backs usually recycle previously ridden terrain. But this part of the Backbone has so many subtleties and technical treats that riding it eastward back to your car is an entirely new, exciting experience. At 12.2 miles you'll be done, thoroughly intoxicated with joy and wishing you brought your night-light so you could do it all over again.

After the Ride

Virtually every international flavor of cuisine can be found on Pacific Coast Highway as you head back to Los Angeles. Cholada Thai Beach Cuisine at 18763 Pacific Coast Highway offers fiery fare as well as cold bottled Thai macrobrews to wash it down; (310) 317-0025. For American food, a full bar, and possibly a musical display from forgotten bands of the 80s, visit The Malibu Inn located across from the historical Malibu Pier at 22969 Pacific Coast Highway; (310) 456-6060.

04

|BULLDOG LOOP

KEY AT-A-GLANCE INFORMATION

Length: 14.6 miles

Configuration: Loop

Technical difficulty: 3

Aerobic difficulty: 5

Scenery: Santa Monica Mountains, Malibu Canyon, Malibu Creek, Castro Peak, Pacific Ocean

Exposure: 70% exposed to sunshine

Trail traffic: Light–moderate on weekdays, moderate–heavy on weekends

Trail surface: Hardpack with embedded rocks, 20% singletrack

Riding time: 2.5–3.5 hours

Access: Sunrise–sunset, 7 days a week

Maps: USGS 7.5-minute quads: Point Dume, Malibu Beach

Special comments: The Bulldog Motorway is a relentless uphill grind; avoid it if you're a novice rider.

GPS TRAILHEAD COORDINATES (WGS84)

UTM Zone   11S

Easting   341896

Northing   3774957

Latitude   N 34.06'13"

Longitude   W 118.42'51"

In Brief

Any utterance of the word "Bulldog" among SoCal local riders will surely elicit groans, sighs, and maybe a warning or two. Climbing the Bulldog Motorway is masochism for all but the most advanced riders but a rewarding challenge nonetheless. Like Sycamore Canyon, Malibu Creek State Park offers plenty of distractions for nonriders and has shorter, less challenging rides, which makes this another great place to drag the whole clan.

Description

Once you've parked on Mulholland Highway like a seasoned local, start this route at the trail entrance off Mulholland, roughly 1,000 feet west of Las Virgenes Road on the south side of Mulholland. After a half mile on this singletrack traverse, you will convene with the oft-traveled and unpaved Crags Drive.

At roughly 1.5 miles, after you pass a body of water called Century Lake—a pond, actually—the trail will evolve from wide, groomed fire road to rocky, technical singletrack, a phenomenon spawned by recent flooding—much to the delight of mountain bikers and hikers. Along this section is a point of historical interest—a location often used for filming the hit TV show *M*A*S*H*. All that remains from that era are a few rusted vehicles.

DIRECTIONS

From Los Angeles, take US 101 North; exit at Las Virgenes Road, and turn left. After about 3.25 miles, turn right on Mulholland Highway; a parking area will appear immediately on your left. If that area is full, you can find additional parking farther down Mulholland Highway on either side of the road on the shoulder.

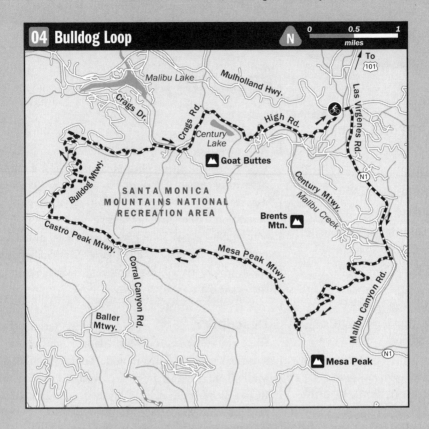

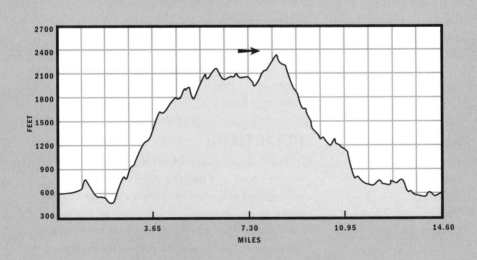

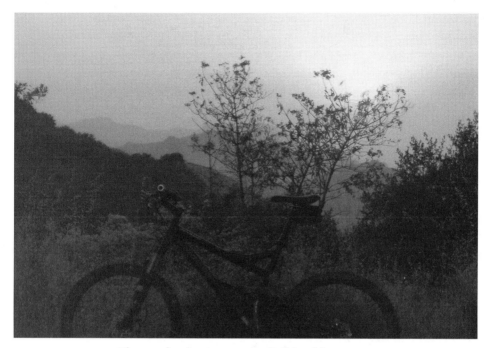

The sun begins to set over Bulldog Motorway.

Let's hope you haven't blown your caloric load by the 3-mile mark because that's the start of the vaunted climb to Castro Peak Motorway via Bulldog Motorway, which involves more than 1,700 feet of climbing over 3 miles of road. Bulldog Motorway is more difficult than the stats suggest because the technical obstacles near the top don't allow for laid-back, in-the-saddle spinning.

After being teased with several false visual impressions of having reached the summit, you'll connect with Castro Peak Motorway roughly 6.4 miles from your car. Although much of the climbing is finished, head back the way you came if your body's spent—the ride ahead is very aerobically demanding.

After a pleasant 1-mile bomb down Castro Peak Motorway, you will see a parking lot at the end of Corral Canyon Road at roughly 7.3 miles from the start. Cross the short lot and follow the singletrack that appears on the left, portaging over the large sandstone rock formations. This 0.4-mile-long section heads east, is very technical, and includes some the longest stretches of slickrock riding to be found in the Santa Monica Mountains. If technical riding like this doesn't suit your fancy, simply go back to the parking lot and head down Corral Canyon Road until it hits Mesa Peak motorway after roughly 0.3 miles, and then turn left.

After evoking visions of Moab, Utah, join Mesa Peak Motorway and ride along a ridge for 2.4 miles with fantastic views of Malibu and the Pacific Ocean to your right, and Malibu Creek State Park to your left. At roughly the 10-mile mark, turn left at the Puerco–Mesa Peak Motorway junction, continuing on Mesa Peak, and start the descent to Las Virgenes Road.

An important right turn comes into view roughly 1.9 miles from the Puerco–Mesa Peak junction, just over 12 miles from the start. Should you fail to make this turn, you will soon encounter a barbed wire fence. If that happens, just backtrack while keeping an eye on your left for a trail entrance. This spur takes you back to Las Virgenes Road after about 0.6 miles. Hang a left and head north on Las Virgenes Road for a slightly uphill mellow 2-mile stretch, and then go left to get back to your car.

Now that you've conquered the infamous Bulldog Motorway, you can either boast your exploits to your pals or be modest and humble, knowing—or pretending—that it was really no big deal. Whatever your impression, 3,300 feet of total elevation gain over 14.73 miles is a big deal and presents a challenge that mountain bikers in flatter states will never ever know.

After the Ride

For margaritas, live music, and Southwestern cuisine, go to the Sagebrush Cantina on 23527 Calabasas Road in Calabasas; (818)-222-6062. For good-quality sushi and sake at a low price, try Tatsuki Restaurant on 21630 Ventura Boulevard in Woodland Hills; (818)-340-8690.

05

CALABASAS PEAK/ COLD CREEK TRAIL

Length: 9.7 miles

Configuration: Out-and-back

Aerobic difficulty: 4

Technical difficulty: 3

Scenery: Views of Saddle Peak, Calabasas, San Fernando Valley, and nearby Santa Monica Mountains and Simi Hills

Exposure: Fully exposed 90%; some shade on Cold Creek Trail

Trail traffic: Light on weekdays, moderate on weekends

Trail surface: 30% singletrack, 70% fire roads; mostly dry and loose, some hardpack

Riding time: 1–2 hours

Access: Sunrise–sunset, 7 days a week

Maps: USGS 7.5-minute quads: Topanga, Calabasas, and Malibu Beach

Special comments: It can be very hot here in summer, so bring plenty of water and use sunblock.

GPS TRAILHEAD
COORDINATES (WGS84)
UTM Zone 11S
Easting 348986
Northing 3775100
Latitude N 34.06'21"
Longitude W 118.37'42"

In Brief

This area is close to many other popular mountain bike destinations in the Santa Monica Mountains, yet it doesn't draw nearly as many fat-tire explorers. Perhaps fewer mountain bikers visit because it is somewhat hard to find, or maybe because it is still largely a secret. Red Rock Canyon offers a phenomenal area for mountain biking, with a unique red-sandstone-addled landscape, clean air, and singletrack that rivals any section of the Backbone Trail.

Description

By the time you reach the parking lot at the end of Red Rock Road, it will be obvious how this area got its name—the sandstone rock formations have a fantastic crimson hue that will remind you of southern Utah if you've been lucky enough to visit there. Unlike southern Utah's, however, these sandstone rocks are for viewing only. Please stay on the trail. The trailhead is easy to find at the west end of the parking lot, continuing where Red Rock Road finished.

The Red Rock Canyon Fire Road starts out flat, paralleling a small creek. There are many large rock formations on both sides of the trail that make for

DIRECTIONS

From Los Angeles, take CA 10 west until it becomes CA 1. Stay on CA 1 for 5.4 miles, and then turn right on Topanga Canyon Road. After 4.3 miles, turn left on Old Topanga Canyon Road, and then turn left on Red Rock Road. The parking lot is at the end of this partially paved road, about 0.8 miles from its start. If coming from the San Fernando Valley, you can reach Red Rock Road by going south on Mulholland Drive from US 101 for 0.5 miles. Then, turn right on Valmar Road, make another right on Mulholland Highway, and make a quick left onto Old Topanga Canyon Road. Continue 3.8 miles to Red Rock Road, on your right.

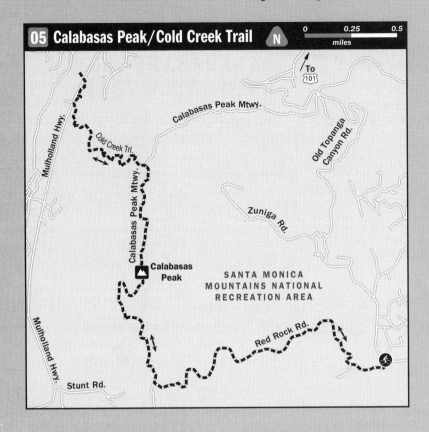

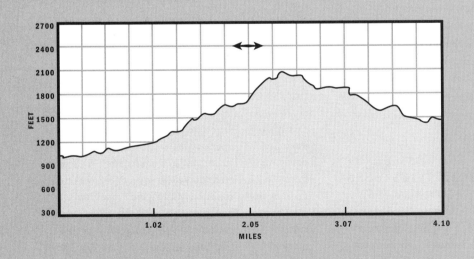

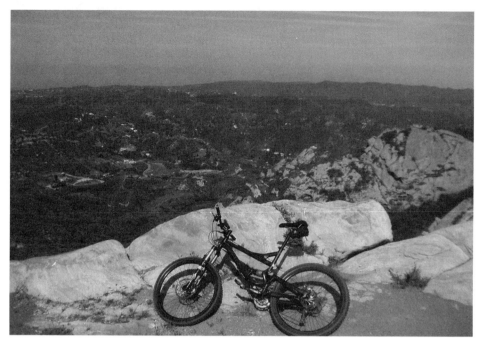

Old Topanga Canyon viewed from Calabasas Peak

such interesting hiking and climbing that you may want to bring an extra pair of suitable shoes. If you have the right gear, stop, indulge, and make this a multiactivity excursion. Back on your bike, the trail becomes steeper and more grueling the farther you go.

Red Rock Canyon Fire Road comes to a T after 1.2 miles and joins Calabasas Peak Fire Road. This section also features a humbling uphill grind, but hopefully the Martian topography will distract you from your burning thighs—a couple of stretches are difficult to pedal even with the granny gear. Remain vigilant and try not to dab so you can preserve momentum. After a mile, you will be somewhat bushed, so stop and have a breather and a snack at Calabasas Peak, which provides great 360-degree views of Saddle Peak, Stunt Road, Topanga Canyon, and the somewhat-less-picturesque San Fernando Valley.

After your picnic, continue north on the fire road and descend to the entrance to the Calabasas/Cold Creek Trail, which is marked by a sign roughly 0.7 miles from Calabasas Peak. When you start this tight singletrack ascent, you'll immediately understand why this route is such a gem. Several stepped switchbacks on this 1.25-mile-long stretch to the end at Mulholland Highway will test your technical skill, but don't worry—the fun's not over. This trail is as much of a joy to ascend as it is to descend.

When you return to the Calabasas Peak Fire Road, turn right to begin the rest of this splendid out-and-back experience with a short climb to Calabasas Peak followed by a blistering plunge back to the trailhead. This descent's speed makes up for any lack of technicality, proving that downhill mountain biking doesn't require technical terrain. Drifting around corners with your foot scraping terra firma is just as much fun as plunking over rocks and catching air, but keep an eye out for equestrian and hiker traffic on your way down.

06

|SANTA MARIA TRAIL

KEY AT-A-GLANCE INFORMATION

Length: 9.5 miles

Configuration: Loop

Technical difficulty: 4

Aerobic difficulty: 3

Scenery: Topanga Canyon, Eagle Peak, Eagle Rock, Santa Ynez Canyon

Exposure: 100% exposed to sunshine

Trail traffic: Light on weekdays, light to moderate on weekends

Trail surface: Dry hardpack with embedded sandstone boulders, some slickrock

Riding time: 1.5–2.5 hours

Access: Sunrise–sunset, 7 days a week

Maps: USGS 7.5-minute quads: Topanga, Canoga Park

Special comments: Heat can be a factor on this ride, so bring lots of water.

In Brief

Although Topanga Canyon is a well-known local destination for LA mountain bikers, much of this nearly 10-mile loop is off the beaten path and known to few. It offers splendid views of Santa Maria Creek and its rock formations, and has the most technical stretch of trail in the area.

Description

From the intersection of Cheney Drive and Topanga Canyon Boulevard, take a 0.6-mile-long spin north up Topanga Canyon Boulevard. The unmarked trailhead starts on the right (east) side of the road, across from Pat's Topanga Grill, on the left (west) side of the road.

The first quarter mile of the trail is a steep lung burner, with just enough traction to keep the strongest riders from having to dab their feet. At roughly 0.25 miles from the trailhead, turn left onto Santa Maria Trail, a well-beaten path. The next 0.4 miles are a mildly ascending singletrack. For those keen on exploration, the famed Santa Maria caves lie amid the large rock formations across Santa Maria Creek, to your right and below where you are riding.

Continue up the trail, mindfully avoiding one descending right turn, and join the paved Santa Maria Road. Ignore any PRIVATE ROAD signs, and spin your way up the gentle, picturesque, albeit asphalt-crusted ascent to unpaved Mulholland Drive. Turn right, go around the

GPS TRAILHEAD COORDINATES (WGS84)

UTM Zone   11S
Easting   353244
Northing   3776687
Latitude   N 34.07'15"
Longitude   W 118.35'29"

DIRECTIONS

From US 101, exit Topanga Canyon Boulevard south. Continue on Topanga Canyon about 6.2 miles until you reach Cheney Drive. Park on the shoulder of the road near this intersection. From Pacific Coast Highway, drive north on Topanga Canyon Boulevard about 6.5 miles until you reach Cheney Drive, and then park on the shoulder.

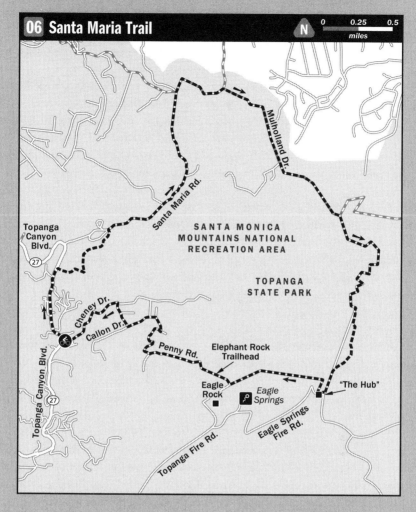

N

0   0.25   0.5
miles

Topanga
Canyon
Blvd.

27

Santa Maria Rd.

SANTA MONICA
MOUNTAINS NATIONAL
RECREATION AREA

Mulholland Dr.

TOPANGA
STATE PARK

Cheney Dr.

Callon Dr.

Topanga Canyon Blvd.

27

Penny Rd.

Elephant Rock
Trailhead

Eagle
Rock

Eagle
Springs

"The Hub"

Eagle Springs
Fire Rd.

Topanga Fire Rd.

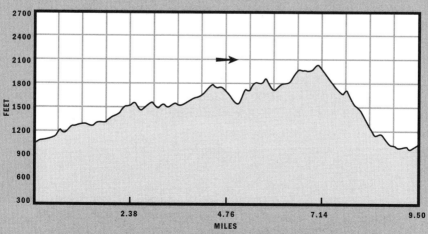

closed gate, and start pedaling on the equally scenic, unpaved, off-limits-to-cars Mulhol-land. On a clear day, you will see the whole San Fernando Valley, along with the Simi Hills and western San Gabriel Mountains. After nearly 2 miles of mellow ascending and descending, turn right on the broad fire road that reenters Topanga State Park.

After about 0.6 miles of easy descending, start the 1.4-mile ascent to "The Hub" or "Hub Junction," the intersection of Eagle Rock Trail, Eagle Springs Trail, and Temescal Ridge Fire Road. From this four-way intersection, turn right, heading northeast on Eagle Rock Trail, which starts with a short ascent. The additional half mile of mild descending will reward you with a great view at Eagle Peak—the gargantuan ancient monolith called Eagle Rock, Santa Ynez Canyon, and possibly the Pacific on a fog-free day.

Treat yourself to full compensation for your aerobic efforts by descending Eagle Rock Trail for 0.4 miles. This stretch could be described as either a narrow fire road or a wide singletrack, but you'll enjoy it even if you're of the "glass is half empty" persuasion because it is fast, steep, and rich in technical subtleties like loose rocks and rain ruts. When this hill flattens out, after roughly 7 miles of riding, turn right and start descending "Elephant Rock Trail"—as it is called by the locals—which is narrow, rutted, and composed mostly of embedded sandstone. About halfway down this 0.6-mile singletrack, a large rock formation with a few caves will appear on the left. Try to figure out why it was given the name "Elephant Rock"—I'm still baffled.

After some amateur spelunking, backtrack a little on the trail, lower your seat, and attempt the remaining descent without dabbing, crashing, or both. You will find it very tough to follow an error-free line on the way down. Don't hesitate to turn around and take a few more runs—you spent a lot of money on your full-suspension rig, so you should see what it can do.

Once you're done goofing around and back on your bike engaging in downward loco-motion, you'll find the trail ends at a fence, beyond which is a private residence. Don't worry—you're not trespassing as long as you go down the driveway. To get back to your car, just follow the road downhill. At the 8.3-mile mark, turn right onto Cheney Drive, and follow this road back to Topanga Canyon Boulevard, at which point your odometer will have hit the 9-mile mark. Give yourself a pat on the back for having faith in local knowledge and the courage to stray off the beaten path. As they say, "When in Topanga . . ."

After the Ride

For a slice of pizza and beer on tap, visit Rocco's in the Canyon, at 123 South Topanga Canyon Boulevard; (310) 455-2487. For Mexican food and an even larger selection of beverages, try Abuelita's Mexican Restaurant at 137 South Topanga Canyon Boulevard; (310) 455-8788.

07

Length: 5.5 miles

Configuration: Loop with partial out-and-back

Technical difficulty: 2

Aerobic difficulty: 2

Scenery: Topanga Canyon, Santa Ynez Canyon, San Fernando Valley

Exposure: 90% exposed to sunshine

Trail traffic: Heavy on weekdays and weekends

Trail surface: Dry, hard-packed fire roads—no singletrack

Riding time: 1.5–2.5 hours

Access: Sunrise–sunset, 7 days a week

Maps: USGS 7.5-minute quad: Topanga

Special comments: Parking is $4 at Trippet Ranch. Free parking on the street helps you avoid being locked in after sunset.

GPS TRAILHEAD COORDINATES (WGS84)

UTM Zone   11S
Easting   353592
Northing   3773624
Latitude   N 34.05'35"
Longitude   W 118.35'13"

EAGLE ROCK/ EAGLE SPRINGS LOOP

In Brief

The Eagle Rock/Eagle Springs Loop, a relatively manageable climb, provides a great place to turn novice riders on to the sport of mountain biking as well as a fun route for experienced riders with limited time. This ride includes a visit to Eagle Rock, perhaps the premier geological wonder of the Santa Monica Mountains.

Description

The trailhead, at the southeastern end of the parking lot, starts with a short, steep climb of about 400 feet, after which the trail joins a fire road. Turn left here, and spin your way up to another junction where you have two choices: either go south to the Parker Mesa overlook, or head north to Eagle Rock. Because the former will be included in another, more challenging route, hang a left now and head up toward Eagle Rock.

Even though the next 1.2 miles of groomed fire road have virtually zero technical subtleties, they aren't easy for beginners because of the roughly 550-foot elevation gain. The pain relents with a few flat spots and minor descents along the way. At 1.4 miles from the start, after a small descent, go left at the fork

DIRECTIONS

From the San Fernando Valley, take US 101 to Topanga Canyon Boulevard and continue toward the ocean (south) for 8 miles. Turn left onto Entrada Road, go 0.7 miles, and then make a left onto Colina Road; go 0.3 miles, and then take another left on Entrada Road. The driveway for Trippet Ranch is 0.1 mile farther on the right. From LA, take CA 10 to Pacific Coast Highway. After 5.4 miles, turn right onto Topanga Canyon Boulevard; continue 4.7 miles, turn right onto Entrada Road, and follow the directions above to reach Trippet Ranch.

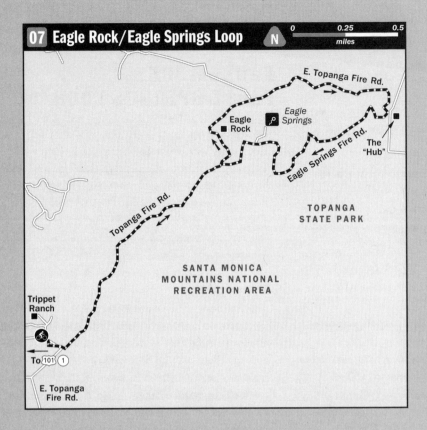

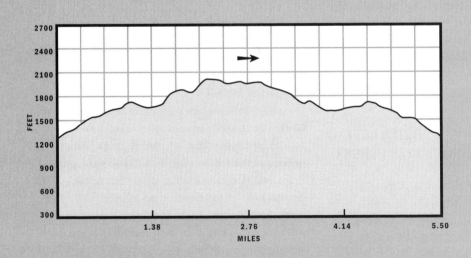

and head up toward Eagle Rock, which is in full view to the north. This is the most challenging section of the route—the trail is almost narrow enough to qualify as singletrack, and there are enough embedded rocks and ruts to make pedaling without dabbing over the next half mile a tricky proposition for the newbie rider.

At about 1.8 miles, you'll round the back side of Eagle Rock, and a short trail will appear on your right leading to a picnic table atop a small hill. Go up the hill, park your steed, and walk to the top of Eagle Rock, where you can enjoy views of Eagle Springs, Santa Ynez Canyon, and the blue Pacific on a clear day. You will find a few caves to goof around in, but don't get too close to the edge with your slippery cycling shoes—the very long drop has claimed victims in the past.

After communing with nature, go back to your g-ride and continue up the fire road until you reach Eagle Peak, roughly 2.4 miles from the start. After this, it's a half-mile trot to "The Hub," as the locals call it, which joins Temescal Ridge Fire Road and leads to Eagle Rock and Eagle Springs Trail. Here you'll find a bulletin board, trash can, and portable toilet.

At this junction, descend Eagle Springs Trail, heading west. Newbies will love this descent because it has long, wide turns and never gets steep enough to warrant nervousness or heavy braking. After 3.9 miles, the blazing descent will end, and you'll pass the natural spring (on the right) for which this trail was named. From the springs, a short ascent returns you to familiar ground as the path rejoins Eagle Rock Trail.

The descent to Trippet Ranch often sees multitudes of hikers making the pilgrimage to Eagle Rock, the most popular hiking destination in the area. After getting to the bottom without scaring any hikers, pat your newbie riding partner (or yourself, for that matter) on the back for completing the route.

After the Ride

The closest culinary attractions to Red Rock Canyon are in Topanga Canyon. For great pizza and beer on tap, visit Rocco's in the Canyon, at 123 South Topanga Canyon Boulevard; (310) 455-2487. For Mexican food and an even larger selection of beverages, try Abuelita's Mexican Restaurant, at 137 South Topanga Canyon Boulevard; (310) 455-8788.

08

PASEO MIRAMAR/EAGLE ROCK/TEMESCAL RIDGE/ TRAILER CANYON LOOP

KEY AT-A-GLANCE INFORMATION

Length: 17.3 miles

Configuration: Loop

Aerobic difficulty: 5

Technical difficulty: 2

Scenery: Santa Monica Bay, Topanga Canyon, Santa Ynez Canyon

Exposure: 90% exposed to sunshine

Trail traffic: Busy

Trail surface: Hard-packed fire roads and pavement— 0% singletrack

Riding time: 2.5–3.5 hours

Access: Sunrise–sunset, 7 days a week

Maps: USGS 7.5-minute quad: Topanga

Special comments: Excessive sun exposure and exhaustion can be a factor here, so bring plenty of H_2O and sunblock.

GPS TRAILHEAD COORDINATES (WGS84)

UTM Zone 11S
Easting 356279
Northing 3768890
Latitude N 34.03'03"
Longitude W 118.33'26"

In Brief

The Paseo Miramar/Parker Mesa/Eagle Rock/Trailer Canyon Loop isn't very technical, but it provides approximately 4,350 feet of total climbing, making it the ideal nearby calorie burner for residents or visitors to West Los Angeles. Since the toughest climbing is just a hop, skip, and jump away from that giant AC unit called the Pacific Ocean, it's tough to overheat on this ride, even on the hottest days of summer.

Description

Compared with the other rides in this book, this one includes a substantial amount of pavement riding—about 38 percent of the total mileage—but the pavement sees light traffic, so you won't be inhaling too much carbon monoxide. Plus, the longest stretch off pavement comes at the end of the ride as you descend the lovely Santa Ynez Canyon via Palisades Drive, making it a scenic experience rather than a tour through urban wasteland.

To minimize time spent in Babylon, this route is designed to keep you rolling downhill on the tarmac, which is why you will be parking at the bottom of Palisades Drive. From there, gear up and ride downhill toward the beach on Sunset Boulevard, keeping an eye out for Paseo Miramar, which will appear on your right roughly 0.14 miles down Sunset. Then let the games begin! The first mile of the pavement is a grueling tour through a

DIRECTIONS

To start this ride, park anywhere along Palisades Drive, in Pacific Palisades. To get there, drive north on Pacific Coast Highway from the Maclure Tunnel about 4.1 miles to Sunset Boulevard. Drive up Sunset about a half mile, and then turn left on Palisades Drive.

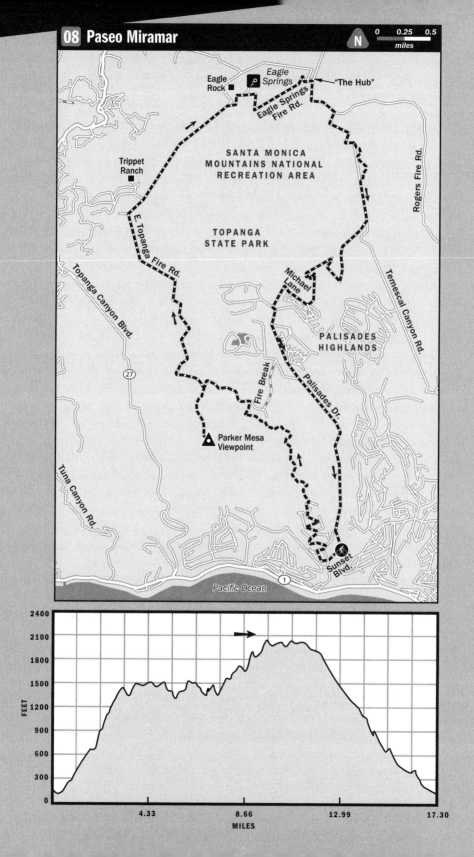

0   0.25   0.5
miles

N

Eagle Rock

Eagle Springs

"The Hub"

Eagle Springs Fire Rd.

Rogers Fire Rd.

SANTA MONICA
MOUNTAINS NATIONAL
RECREATION AREA

Trippet Ranch

TOPANGA
STATE PARK

E. Topanga Fire Rd.

Michael Lane

Temescal Canyon Rd.

Topanga Canyon Blvd.

27

PALISADES
HIGHLANDS

Fire Break

Palisades Dr.

Parker Mesa
Viewpoint

Tuna Canyon Rd.

Sunset Blvd.

1

Pacific Ocean

2400
2100
1800
1500
1200
900
600
300
0

FEET

4.33   8.66   12.99   17.30

MILES

plethora of fancy SoCal real estate. The fragrance emanating from the meticulously maintained gardens will kill the nauseating bouquet from the exhaust system of the occasional gas-guzzling luxury SUV that passes you on the way up.

You should be thoroughly drenched in sweat and ready to rock when you reach the entrance to the unpaved portion Paseo Miramar. Don't rush it—you've got more than 800 feet of elevation to gain in the next 2 miles, so favor the bigger cogs on your cassette and possibly the granny gear of your crankset, and pace yourself. At about 4 miles from your car, hang a left at the first junction that comes into view—a short spur to the Parker Mesa Overlook, which is signposted. An absence of the marine fog that the locals call "May gray" or "June gloom" (although it can blanket the ocean any month of the year) will reveal the expanse of Santa Monica Bay, Palos Verdes, Santa Catalina Island, and possibly the distant hump of land called Santa Barbara Island. A recently installed picnic bench is the prime perch for admiring this vista, and a great place to replenish your essential fuels.

After your break, retrace your steps along the spur and turn left where Paseo Miramar ends and the Santa Ynez Fire Road originates. The next 2.5 miles is a nice up-and-down sprintable section, with two items of great scenic interest—the lower, unpopulated reaches of Topanga Canyon on your left, which served as an illegitimate camping area for wandering hippies in the 1960s, and Santa Ynez Canyon on your right. (An interesting footnote: somewhere amid the towering sycamores and oaks down to your left lies the infamous "Twin Poles" hippie settlement of Topanga Canyon—the stomping grounds of Charles Manson before he gained national notoriety.) Interestingly, the populace that settled the areas to your left also stood on the left side of the political spectrum, as did the very un-Bohemian suburbanites to your right, in the Pacific Palisades.

Your traverse along the center line of this area's landscape reaches a well-marked junction, which can take you to one of the bases of the park-ranger bureaucracy called Trippet Ranch, which includes a small museum exhibit and murals with historical info and factoids about the natural wonders of the area, as well as barbecues, park facilities, and a small pond. On this journey, you'll avoid that off-ramp and continue up the hill toward Eagle Rock. The ascent to Eagle Rock is less excruciating than the climb up Paseo Miramar, but 550 feet of gain over 1.7 miles is no picnic, so pace yourself here as well.

At 1.3 miles from the Santa Ynez–Trippet Ranch junction, avoid navigational mishap by turning left on the only fork that appears in this area so you can spin your way up the most technical and steep part of the ride toward Eagle Rock. This gigantic hunk of Swiss cheese is the premier natural wonder of the Santa Monica Mountains. The climb will display this great rock and then take you around the backside of it, but don't worry—at 1.7 miles from the Trippet Ranch turnoff (roughly 9 miles from your car), a trail will appear on your right that will allow you to dismount, hike to the top of the rock, and explore its caves and other surface subtleties as well as peer down at the picturesque Santa Ynez Canyon below. This site gains its namesake probably because it served as a great perch for the native predator called the red-tailed hawk before *Homo sapiens* took over.

After some transcendental meditation atop Eagle Rock, return to your steel, alloy, or carbon steed and continue up the fire road to Hub junction. At this intersection of three fire roads, you will be trampling the same dirt that legends such as Tinker Juarez, Victor Vincente, and Brian Skinner—key figures in the genesis of mountain biking—have ridden. "The Hub" also served as the midpoint of the sport's earliest competitive event: the "Reseda to the Sea" race, organized by Vincente, who rode it on his very own 20-inch-wheeled custom bike, the "Topanga," one of the first mountain bikes ever manufactured.

Leave this piece of mountain bike history and ride south along Temescal Ridge about 3 miles, and then turn right to descend the Trailer Canyon Fire Road, which drops down into Santa Ynez Canyon. The corners on this road will test your drifting skills, but watch out for the numerous apple-sized rocks that can easily make things interesting. The dirt ends about 14.3 miles from your start, dumping you into the suburban splendor of the Palisades Highlands. To get back to your car, just go downhill, making a right turn on Michael Lane and then a quick left at the end, followed by a right on Palisades Drive. Tuck down low to decrease your drag coefficient, and you'll be back at your car in no time, forgetting that you committed the cardinal sin of riding on pavement for more than a mile.

After the Ride

For an excellent slice of pizza, plus salads and fountain drinks, go to Rocco's Cucina at 17338 West Sunset Boulevard; (310) 573-3727. For seafood and beers on tap with ocean views, go to Gladstone's Restaurant at 17300 Pacific Coast Highway; (310) 573-3727.

09

KEY AT-A-GLANCE INFORMATION

Length: 13.7 miles

Configuration: Out-and-back

Technical difficulty: 3

Aerobic difficulty: 4

Scenery: Rustic Canyon, Temescal Canyon, Santa Ynez Canyon

Exposure: 80% exposed to sunshine

Trail traffic: Light–moderate weekdays, moderate–heavy weekends

Trail surface: Mostly hard-packed and dry with embedded rocks—90% singletrack

Riding time: 2.5–3.5 hours

Access: Sunrise–sunset, 7 days a week

Maps: USGS 7.5-minute quad: Topanga

Special comments: Excessive heat, poison oak, and sun exposure present potential hazards on this ride.

GPS TRAILHEAD COORDINATES (WGS84)

UTM Zone   11S
Easting   360461
Northing   3769463
Latitude   N 34.03'24"
Longitude   W 118.30'43"

BACKBONE TRAIL: WILL ROGERS SHP TO TEMESCAL RIDGE

In Brief

So, you want to ride singletrack, but you're not willing or don't have the time to drive to a far away destination? If that's the case, go to Will Rogers State Historic Park (SHP) and ride the southernmost end of the Backbone Trail. It's within 10 miles of Santa Monica, Culver City, Beverly Hills, Hollywood, Sherman Oaks, and Encino. With 3,570 feet of total elevation gain, this ride features a startlingly high degree of aerobic difficulty.

Description

The fact that this section of the Backbone Trail is still open despite being in the backyard of many wealthy and powerful hikers and equestrians is nothing short of a miracle. This 7-mile-long singletrack has been designated a multiuse trail, which means it is open to humans, humans on horseback, and humans on bikes. The only rule you need to remember is that you need to yield to hikers and horseback riders at all times, and that is crucial on this trail because there are people who could probably have mountain bikers banned from the area with one simple phone call to their personal friend, the governor of California.

Before you get started on the ride, please stop and take in your surroundings. Long ago, the famous humorist and Hollywood actor Will Rogers made this place his

DIRECTIONS

From the San Fernando Valley, head south (if coming from Los Angeles, head north) on I-405. Take the Sunset Boulevard exit and drive west (toward the ocean). Continue 4.4 miles on Sunset, and turn right onto Will Rogers State Park Road. Take this road 1 mile until it terminates at the parking area at Will Rogers State Historic Park. The trailhead is just north of the polo field.

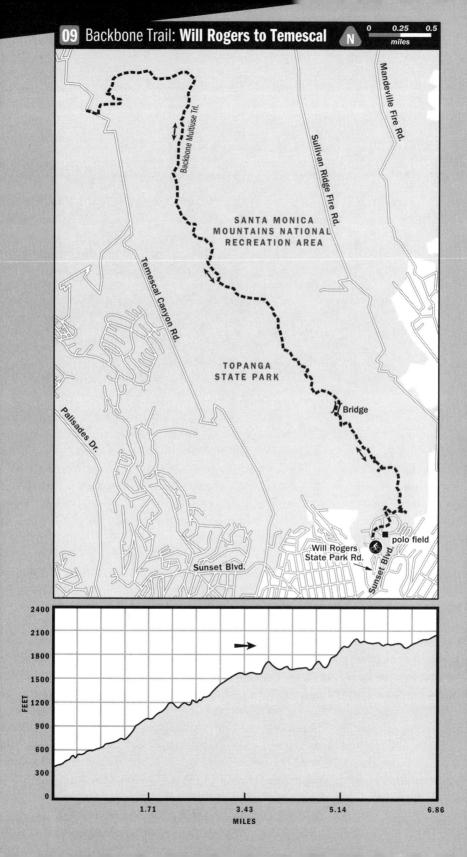

N

0   0.25   0.5
miles

Backbone Multiuse Trl.

Sullivan Ridge Fire Rd.

Mandeville Fire Rd.

SANTA MONICA
MOUNTAINS NATIONAL
RECREATION AREA

Temescal Canyon Rd.

TOPANGA
STATE PARK

Bridge

Palisades Dr.

polo field

Will Rogers
State Park Rd.

Sunset Blvd.

Sunset Blvd.

FEET

2400
2100
1800
1500
1200
900
600
300
0

1.71   3.43   5.14   6.86
MILES

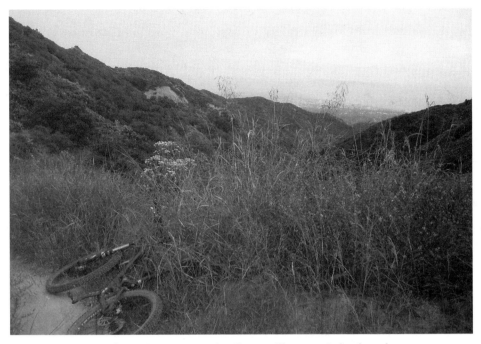

Looking at Santa Monica from Will Rogers's backyard

personal playground, where he and his pals could pursue their favorite pastimes—riding horses, roping, golf, and polo—until Rogers's unfortunate death in a plane crash. Now his estate is a public park, so you don't have to be in the social circle of LA's billionaires to hang out, but you'll have to leave thoughts of sunbathing on the grass with Ginger Rogers beneath the overhead buzzing of one of Howard Hughes's private jets to your imagination. If mountain bikes had been around in the early 1930s, Will Rogers would have been stoked because he had some great singletrack on his private property.

After checking your work e-mail in the parking lot (the park is now a Wi-Fi hot spot), mount up and ride eastward along the parking lot to ascend the road that borders the east side of the golf course. Hang a right at the northern end of the golf course and go up the eucalyptus-lined dirt road to the start of the Backbone Multiuse Trail, marked by a clearly visible sign.

The first 2 miles of the trail are the toughest, so keep your bike in granny gear to avoid seizing your engines. The several wooden steps provide a tough technical challenge because they require you accelerate on steep hills if you want to ride over them without stopping. About 2.5 miles from your car, you'll see a sign that orders all bicyclists to dismount and walk. This is not a suggestion: submit to authority and walk your bike over the short bridge and subsequent steep switchback just beyond; you are walking your bike to minimize damage to the old bridge and trail erosion. Another sign will inform you when you can remount after the switchback. This is the last piece of red tape you'll encounter on this route (until you recross the bridge on your return).

The aerobic toughness subsides after nearly 3 miles, when a large oak tree appears in the trail. As all the trampled ground around the oak suggests, this place marks the point at which most mortals turn around and head back. Since you're not the average sissy, keep on trucking. The trail gets less and less steep as you progress. The next 2.5 miles will see less than half the elevation gain of the first 3 miles, but there will be plenty of overgrowth impeding your progress. Although it receives an occasional grooming, this area has heavy poison-oak growth, so be wary.

At about 5.7 miles, come to a fork in the trail and go left to complete the southernmost section of the Backbone. This nicely groomed 1.3-mile stretch has a thick foliage canopy above, making it seem like a tunnel at times. At the end, the Backbone intersects with the Temescal Ridge Fire Road. Take a rest here.

The return ride to Will Rogers SHP rewards you for all your hard work; the 6-plus miles of continuous singletrack descent are well worth it. As long as there's no fog, you will be looking straight at the Santa Monica Pier as you descend. Have fun, be responsible, and please remember to dismount at the bridge.

After the Ride

For a great selection of Mexi-Cali platters, vegetarian dishes, and burgers, head to Kay and Dave's Fresh Mex Cantina at 15246 Sunset Boulevard in Pacific Palisades; (310)-459-8118. If you're a little more thirsty, try the Pearl Dragon, which boasts a full bar and Asian-fusion vittles, at 15229 West Sunset Boulevard in Pacific Palisades; (310)-459-9790.

KEY AT-A-GLANCE INFORMATION

Length: 13.5 miles

Configuration: Figure-8

Difficulty: Moderate

Scenery: Fantastic views of San Fernando Valley, San Gabriel Mountains, downtown Los Angeles, Santa Monica Bay, and Catalina Island

Exposure: Sunny on Sullivan Ridge and "MG" singletrack, shady in Sullivan Canyon

Trail traffic: Moderate on weekdays, heavy on weekends

Trail surface: Fire roads and singletrack

Riding time: 2–3 hours

Access: Free for day use

Maps: USGS quad: Topanga

Special comments: Please be wary of hikers and dog walkers—there are many on this route. Yield to them as required.

GPS TRAILHEAD COORDINATES (WGS84)

UTM Zone   11 S
Easting   360790
Northing   3772263
Latitude   N 34.05'08"
Longitude   W 118.30'32"

SULLIVAN RIDGE TO SULLIVAN CANYON LOOP WITH "MG" SINGLETRACK

In Brief

Despite being so close to West Los Angeles, this route provides some of the best scenery and singletrack action that the Santa Monica Mountains National Recreation Area has to offer. The technical and aerobic difficulty is moderate, but novice riders may find themselves winded early—a simple out-and-back up Sullivan Canyon or to the Nike Missile Base via the West Mandeville Fire Road (known locally as Westridge) may be more desirable than riding the full length of the described route.

Description

To best enjoy the terrain, mount up at the entrance to the Sullivan Ridge Fire Road. You'll find ample parking here, even on the busiest days, so if the small lot is full, simply find street parking anywhere on Westridge Road. Lacking exceptionally steep sections, the Sullivan Ridge Fire Road provides a great warm-up for this ride; each small climb is followed by a level section or descent that allows the rusty rider to cool down. As you ascend the ridge, you will notice a singletrack that parallels and meanders across both sides of the fire road. If the fire road's predictable features and lack of technical difficulty are too dull for you, switch over to the singletrack.

DIRECTIONS

From the San Fernando Valley, head south (if coming from Los Angeles, head north) on I-405. Take the Sunset Boulevard exit, and drive west (toward the ocean). Continue on Sunset Boulevard 2.37 miles, and then turn right onto Mandeville Canyon Road. Continue on Mandeville Canyon for 0.25 miles, and then turn left onto Westridge Road. Stay on Westridge Road 2.23 miles until you reach a dead end, which is the Sullivan Ridge trailhead and parking lot.

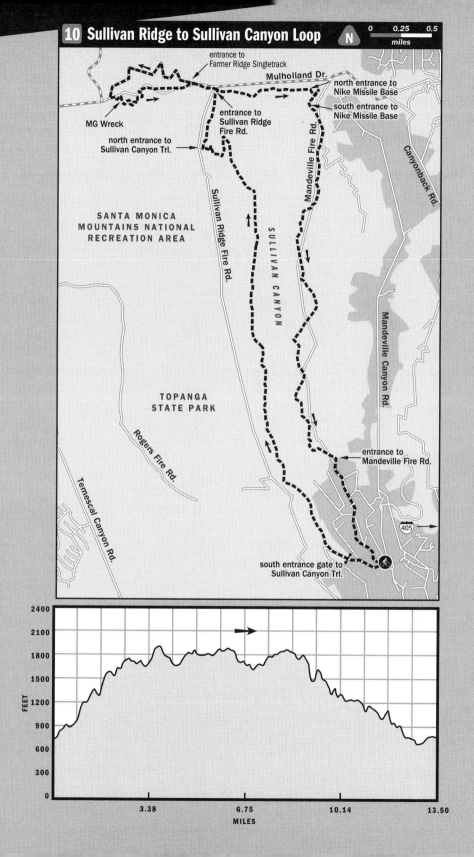

N

0   0.25   0.5
miles

entrance to
Farmer Ridge Singletrack

Mulholland Dr.

north entrance to
Nike Missile Base

south entrance to
Nike Missile Base

entrance to
Sullivan Ridge
Fire Rd.

MG Wreck

north entrance to
Sullivan Canyon Trl.

Mandeville Fire Rd.

Canyonback Rd.

SANTA MONICA
MOUNTAINS NATIONAL
RECREATION AREA

Sullivan Ridge Fire Rd.

SULLIVAN CANYON

Mandeville Canyon Rd.

TOPANGA
STATE PARK

Rogers Fire Rd.

entrance to
Mandeville Fire Rd.

Tennescal Canyon Rd.

405

south entrance gate to
Sullivan Canyon Trl.

2400					
2100					
1800					
1500					
1200					
900					
600					
300					
0					

FEET

3.38   6.75   10.14   13.50

MILES

At 3.45 miles, you'll reach the Nike Missile Base entrance gate. To fully appreciate this Cold War relic, watch *Dr. Strangelove* the night before the ride. Fortunately, the base has been shut down since the good old days when a Russian long-range bomber attack was the biggest threat to America. Now part of the state park, the base offers picnic tables, restrooms, a drinking fountain, a pay phone, and a coin-operated observation telescope to get a closer look at West LA. Don't forget to bring a quarter!

Continue down the driveway toward the beckoning San Fernando Valley, and exit the facility at its north entrance, which intersects the unpaved portion of Mulholland Drive. Turn left onto Mulholland, and reenter the state park. For the next 1.1 miles, tool along a wide fire road with minimal elevation changes and great views of San Fernando Valley to your right and the Santa Monica Mountains to your left. This area is heavily frequented by hikers and dog walkers—once again, yield at all times. In case the ride sounds a bit tame thus far, don't worry—the pace and difficulty pick up soon.

A little more than a mile beyond the north entrance to the Nike Missile Base on Mulholland Drive, look on your left for a yellow gate marked FARMER RIDGE with a trail behind it going up a small hill. Cross the gate, and for the next 0.4 miles enjoy an ungroomed road that has reverted to singletrack. Stay on the lookout for the entrance to the "MG" singletrack on your left.

Almost immediately, the MG will have you sporting a perma-grin with its roller-coaster-like ups, downs, and sharp turns. Ride slowly and precisely; you could fall a long way at many points on this trail if you were to accidentally ride off the edge. After the first quarter mile on the MG, turn left and briefly merge with Rustic Canyon Trail for about 50 feet; then turn right and return to the MG. Your next landmark is the namesake of this trail: a mangled orange MG coupe resting in a ditch on your left directly below Mulholland Drive.

Given the wildness of the area you're in, it's hard to realize how close you are to one of the largest cities in the world. Continue carefully to the end of the MG singletrack, where you will once again intersect Mulholland Drive. Turn right and head back toward the Nike Missile Base. This section of Mulholland features a steady 1.3-mile climb to the entrance of the West Mandeville (Westridge) Fire Road on your right. Enjoy the views of the San Fernando Valley and the Encino Reservoir to your left before you descend Sullivan Ridge about 0.5 miles. Watch for a trail offshoot on your left and a sign for Sullivan Canyon Trail. This is where the real fun begins.

Courtesy of the floods of 2004, this changeling trail transformed from a wide double-track into an exiting singletrack with plenty of quick turns, ruts, and rocks to get your adrenaline flowing. Unfortunately, the park service has legitimate reasons to occasionally maintain all fire roads, so from time to time they groom and widen them. To the delight of riders, the park service elected to leave the trail alone well into 2007.

The 4.25-mile-long Sullivan Canyon Trail starts off steep and narrow. (Needless to say, downhillers love this section.) Slow down for blind corners, and be aware of hikers and bikers coming up the trail. After a half mile of downhill bliss, begin to parallel Sullivan Creek. Here the trail narrows, with ruts on both sides. Eventually the trail crosses the creek, splits, and then rejoins itself. Fallen trees, small drops, whoops, and creek crossings will test your suspension settings and put a smile on your face. You can choose from two parallel trails at times, providing easier or more-difficult alternative routes. Trail steepness lessens as you progress, becoming nearly level. Although amply shaded by numerous sycamore trees and steep canyon walls, Sullivan Canyon lacks exposure to the cool ocean breezes in summer. If you ride this trail between June and October, be sure to bring enough fluids to stay hydrated.

The Sullivan Canyon Trail widens to fire-road width before terminating approximately 4.25 miles from its intersection with the Sullivan Ridge Fire Road. Turn up the steep paved road going left, which is approximately an eighth-mile long and leads to the south entrance of Sullivan Canyon Trail.

The rest of the ride is a short pavement excursion back to the trailhead. After you cross the gate onto Queensferry Road, turn right onto Bayliss Road to return to Westridge Road, where you will turn left and ascend back to your car. If you don't want to end your day with a steep climb, parking on Bayliss to reserve the climb up Westridge as a pre-dirt warm-up.

After the Ride

Sullivan Ridge and Sullivan Canyon are within just a few miles of the Sunset Strip, Beverly Hills, and Santa Monica, so there are literally hundreds of great places to go for a bite to eat after the ride. For a relaxed surrounding, try the world-famous Father's Office pub in Santa Monica (1018 Montana Avenue; [310] 393-2337), which boasts 30 different beers on tap plus gourmet cheeseburgers. Sushi lovers should pay a visit to Sushi Masu, at 1911 Westwood Boulevard in West LA; (310) 446-4368.

KEY AT-A-GLANCE INFORMATION

Length: 11.8 miles

Configuration: Out-and-back

Technical difficulty: 3

Aerobic difficulty: 4

Scenery: Sullivan Canyon, Rustic Canyon, Santa Monica Mountains, San Fernando Valley, West LA

Exposure: 95% exposed to sunshine

Trail traffic: Moderate–heavy

Trail surface: Dry, occasionally loose, hardpack—40% singletrack

Riding time: 1.5–2.5 hours

Access: Sunrise–sunset, 7 days a week

Maps: USGS 7.5-minute quads: Topanga, Canoga Park

Special comments: Area can be hot, so bring plenty of water and sunblock.

GPS TRAILHEAD COORDINATES (WGS84)

UTM Zone   11S
Easting   361123
Northing   377025
Latitude   N 34.03'50"
Longitude   W 118.30'18"

SULLIVAN RIDGE SINGLETRACK

In Brief

The drawing of this route may make it look like an out-and-back; however, it is anything but. It involves a very tough fire-road ascent, followed by a bomb down the singletrack that parallels the fire road. This is the bread-and-butter proving ground of Westside XC riders, affording plenty of aerobic and technical challenges. The ride's centralized location and modest length make it an ideal alternative to visiting a sweaty, crowded gym after work.

Description

Once you've found parking somewhere along Capri Road, mount up, climb the end of Capri, and turn left onto Casale Road. After a short spin on pavement, go around the yellow gate and continue up Sullivan Ridge Fire Road. The spooky old gate on your left marks the boundaries of an abandoned neighborhood of estates in the depths of Rustic Canyon. Urban legends and hearsay tell of a group of Nazi sympathizers who once lived here. Whether the story is true or not, the creepy rundown homes are worth a look-see; you can access them via the main driveway or by descending the labyrinthine stairways and paths that traverse the large property. Local downhillers sometimes ride down the "Scares," a very steep, narrow, concrete

DIRECTIONS

From the San Fernando Valley, head south (if coming from Los Angeles, head north) on I-405. Take the Sunset Boulevard exit, and drive west (toward the ocean). Continue on Sunset Boulevard for about 3 miles, and then turn right onto Capri Drive. After 0.3 miles, go around the cul-de-sac and continue on Capri Drive until it terminates at Casale Road; find a parking spot. The trailhead is at the west end of Casale Road, roughly an eighth of a mile from the end of Capri Drive, but you'll have to park off Capri because parking on Casale is prohibited.

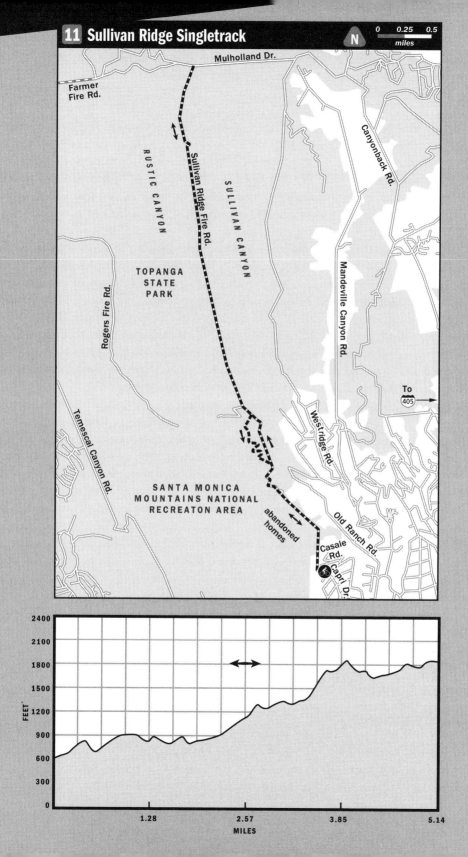

0   0.25   0.5
miles

N

Mulholland Dr.

Farmer
Fire Rd.

Canyonback Rd.

R U S T I C   C A N Y O N

Sullivan Ridge Fire Rd.

S U L L I V A N   C A N Y O N

Mandeville Canyon Rd.

TOPANGA
STATE
PARK

Rogers Fire Rd.

To
405

Westridge Rd.

Temescal Canyon Rd.

SANTA MONICA
MOUNTAINS NATIONAL
RECREATON AREA

abandoned
homes

Old Ranch Rd.

Casale
Rd.

Capri Dr.

FEET

2400
2100
1800
1500
1200
900
600
300
0

1.28   2.57   3.85   5.14
MILES

stairway of many hundred steps that leads to the bottom of Rustic Canyon. (Because this location is very dangerous, I've omitted specific directions to it.)

Just under 2 miles beyond the first gate, dirt will replace pavement after a second gate, and you'll be just warm enough at this point to pedal up a monster hill. If it weren't for the flat spots and brief downhills along the way that provide breathers, this would be one of the toughest climbs in SoCal. Nevertheless, about 1,000 feet of elevation gain over 3.5 miles is no walk in the park. Sullivan Ridge lies between two canyons—Rustic Canyon on your left and Sullivan Canyon to your right. The higher reaches of Sullivan Ridge reveal the other two fashionable mountain bike stomping grounds of West LA: the Backbone Trail, which snakes along the next ridge to the west, and Westridge Fire Road on the adjacent ridge to the east. Routes incorporating those trails are discussed elsewhere in this book.

The Sullivan Ridge Fire Road terminates roughly 5.75 miles from your car and 3.5 miles from the end of pavement, intersecting with the unpaved, car-free portion of Mulholland Drive. When you stop and take a breather here, facing north you'll have views of the San Fernando Valley and the mountains beyond, as well as the unnatural body of water that is the Encino Reservoir. Turn around and head back down the Sullivan Ridge Fire Road. As you start to descend, a profound sense of freedom and excitement will take over because you have many options ahead. Less technically skilled (or mellow) riders will prefer an easy blast down the fire road back to point A. The more adventurous bunch should definitely exploit the singletrack that snakes and parallels the fire road on the way up.

The first singletrack section parallels the first mile. A unique and sometimes perilous type of geology will be making contact with your knobbies here—small, sharp-edged, shalelike rocks that form the crust of the trail. Although they compact nicely and form a stable medium, on the steeper sections they make finding traction a nearly impossible task, so turn your brain into an antilock-braking-system microprocessor and carefully meter out pressure to each brake without skidding.

After the first section, rejoin the main fire road briefly and ride another parallel section. Intersecting singletracks are the trend until 2.25 miles from Mulholland, or about 8 miles from the start, when the next portion of singletrack takes you up a short, steep lung-buster and away from view of the fire road. The next 0.9 miles plummet 600 vertical feet over numerous ruts, all covered in the small, square-edged shaley rocks native to the area. Any failure to keep it "rubber side down" on this route will probably occur on this section.

If you choose to ride the obscenely steep and loose slide back down the fire road to the gate you passed on the way up, do so carefully. Spin on familiar pavement for about 0.2 miles, keeping an eye out for another singletrack offshoot on your right. This section will take you along the hillside below the paved road. The trail composition is more typical here, with loose shale replaced by hard-packed dry clay with embedded sandstones. Overgrowth in the summer can obscure the left turn that takes you back to the road after roughly 0.6 miles, for 10 miles of total riding.

Watch out for dog walkers, joggers, and other bikers as you negotiate the rest of the paved road. Don't forget to visit the spooky estates in Rustic Canyon if you've got time. They are very *Blair Witch Project*. Haunted-house visit excluded, you just completed an 11.5-mile ride with more than 2,200 feet of total elevation gain. Congratulations!

|KENTER WHOOPS

KEY AT-A-GLANCE INFORMATION

Length: 7.6 miles

Configuration: Out-and-back

Technical difficulty: 5

Aerobic difficulty: 3

Scenery: Mandeville Canyon, Santa Monica Mountains, West Los Angeles

Exposure: 95% exposed to sunshine

Trail traffic: Moderate–heavy

Trail surface: Dry hardpack—20% singletrack

Riding time: 1.5–2.5 hours

Access: Sunrise–sunset, 7 days a week

Maps: USGS 7.5-minute quads: Beverly Hills, Topanga

Special comments: This ride is on private property that is open to the public. Wear pads and possibly a full-face helmet if you plan on doing big jumps.

In Brief

The Kenter Whoops are a marvel of human engineering and excavation. Created by local riders over the last 20 years, this 0.9-mile-long roller-coaster ride of whoops and jumps would surely have been bulldozed long ago had it been part of the state park system. Thankfully, the landowners have left this gem alone and have kept the area open to users. Some of the double jumps on this trail are Evel Knievel huge and should be attempted only by experienced dirt jumpers who drape themselves in protective gear. Because of the extreme difficulty, this is by far the most technically demanding ride in the Santa Monica Mountains. However, you don't have to be Brian Lopes to ride here—every double can be ridden around safely.

Description

The Kenter Whoops is a relatively small part of the large riding area located on top of Kenter Ridge. Just riding the whoops alone, although exhilarating, provides very little cardio workout. To afford a complete fat-tire experience, this route includes an extended fire-road climb well beyond the whoops area, as well as some out-and-back action on a little-known piece of singletrack that descends into Mandeville Canyon.

Out of respect for the dirt jumpers who built the whoops, ascend on Kenter Ridge Fire Road instead of going against the grain up the Kenter Whoops trail.

GPS TRAILHEAD COORDINATES (WGS84)
UTM Zone 11S
Easting 362101
Northing 3772233
Latitude N 34.04'54"
Longitude W 118.29'41"

DIRECTIONS

From I-405, exit onto Sunset Boulevard and head west about 1.25 miles. Turn right onto Kenter Avenue and drive to the end, about 2.1 miles from Sunset, and find street parking. The trailhead is clearly marked with a large gate at the end of Kenter.

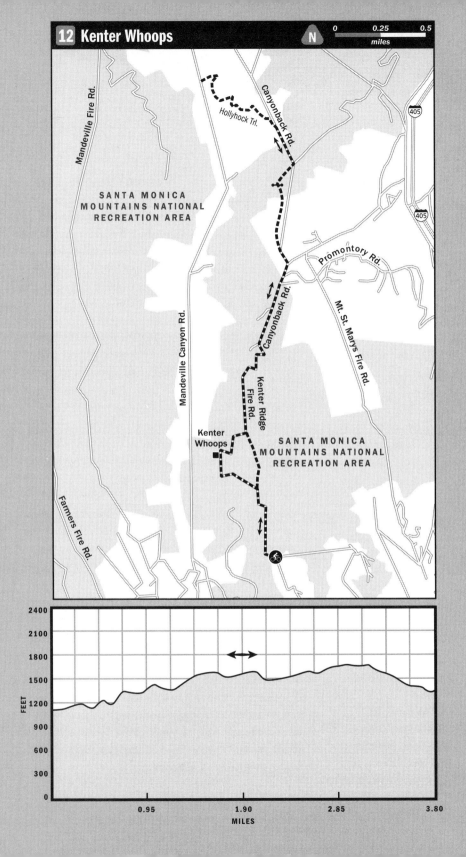

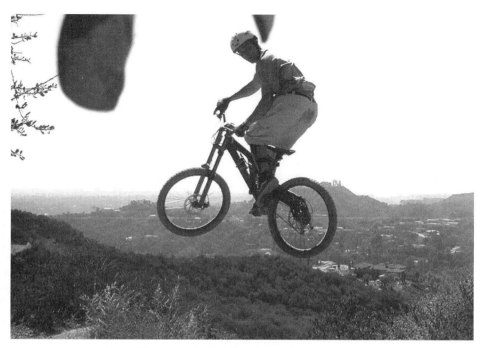

Deker Williams no-looks the gap at the Kenter Whoops.

After roughly 1 mile of moderate climbing, you'll see the entrance to the Kenter Whoops on the left of the trail on the other side of a concrete embankment and small section of fence. There you may see some armor-clad-full-face-helmeted stunt riders straddling their specialized dirt-assaulting bikes. Keep spinning up the ridge; you will join that motley crew later on.

Sweat starts to flow after another mile, and uphill dirt becomes a steep pavement descent with a gate at the bottom. Dismount and step around the gate, and then ride for a half mile on Canyonback Road through an affluent community that one hopes will not edge the Whoops into oblivion through expansion. At the end of Canyonback Road, cross another gate on your left so you can rejoin Kenter Ridge Fire Road and pedal on the raw earth your bike craves. After another half mile of moderate ascending, keep an eye out for an elusive singletrack offshoot on your left. Called Hollyhock Trail by locals, this twisty, seldom-visited descent into Mandeville Canyon was once paved with asphalt. Mother Nature has taken back all but a sliver of this defunct street. Where else would an off-road cyclist enjoy being on pavement?

The Hollyhock singletrack descent is roughly 0.75 miles long, but you will have lost just more than 400 feet of elevation by the time you reach the end at Mandeville Canyon Road, so prepare yourself for a workout when you head back up to Kenter Ridge. Keep the faith, though, salvation is just ahead—you're a few pedal strokes away from the one of the most precious trails in Southern Cali: the Kenter Whoops.

Be sure you lower your seat before you begin bombing down the trail, especially if you plan on doing any aerial stunts. The whoops and jumps on this trail actually began as water bars designed to divert floodwaters down the hillside to prevent trail erosion. The first few whoops aren't very steep or high, so they are an easy initiation into the world of dirt jumping. After about an eighth of a mile, some carefully sculpted steep-faced jumps bob up on either side of the trail. Each jump, called a double, consists of two consecutive humps; the first hump launches you up and, with enough speed, over the second hump. Or you can take it easy and dip up and down both humps, or just take the easier path down the middle. A gifted rider can take off and land on the downward face of the second mound in perfect rhythm. Some of the gaps are more than 20 feet across, so don't try them unless you are very experienced. A little more than a half mile down this virtual motocross track, you'll see some of the most popular doubles, as well as the "Gap," a double jump with a 15-foot-deep gulch between the takeoff and landing. This is a good spot to take a break (out of the way of the riders, of course) and marvel at the skill and grace of jumpers taking precise lines down the trail and fearlessly gliding through the air.

The last quarter mile has a few doubles with 30-plus-foot-long gaps that, believe it or not, have been cleared by a few mortal humans. Like all the obstacles you've seen, these are optional stunts. At the conclusion of the whoops, only disabling injury will keep you from taking another run, so turn left onto Kenter Ridge and begin your laps.

After the Ride

For an eclectic fusion of Asian and Latin cuisines, as well as cheap beer, check out Wahoo's Fish Tacos on 11911 Wilshire Boulevard; (310) 445-5990. For vegan food that even meat eaters love, go to Native Foods on 1110½ Gayley Avenue; (310) 209-1055.

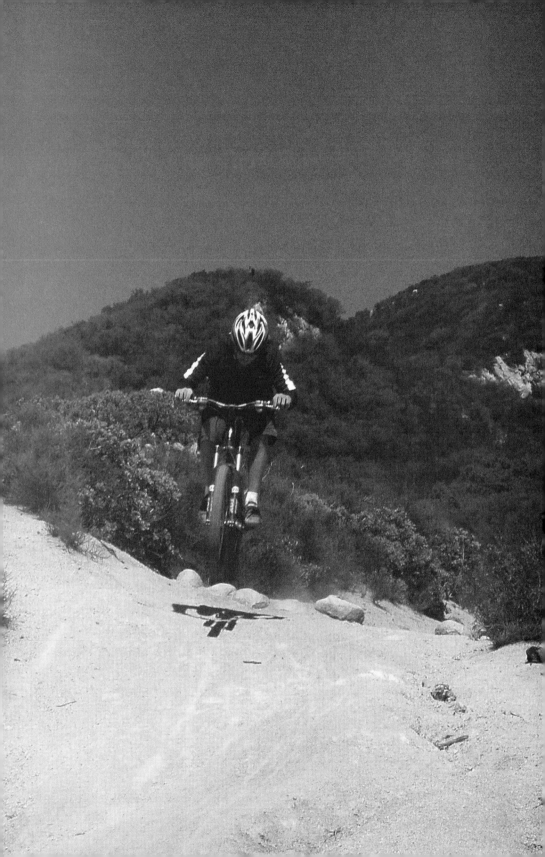

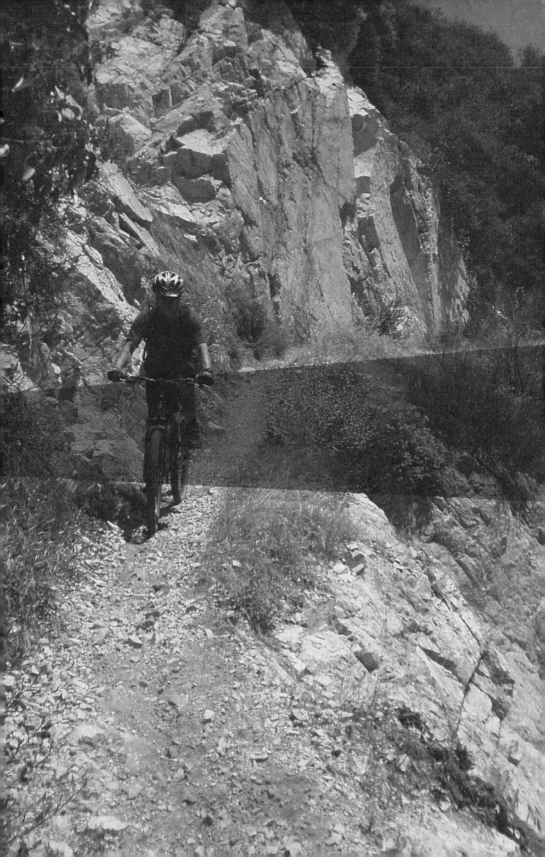

SANTA MONICA MOUNTAINS EAST

13

| LOS ROBLES TRAIL

Length: 7.14 miles

Configuration: Out-and-back

Technical difficulty: 4

Aerobic difficulty: 3

Scenery: Santa Monica Mountains, Thousand Oaks, Simi Peak, Sandstone Peak, Las Posas Hills

Exposure: 70% exposed to sunshine

Trail traffic: Heavy on weekdays and weekends

Trail surface: Hard-packed, dry with embedded and loose rocks— 90% singletrack

Riding time: 1–2 hours

Access: Sunrise–sunset, 7 days a week

Maps: USGS 7.5-minute quad: Newbury Park

Special comments: Watch for heavy trail traffic around blind turns.

In Brief

You may want to move to Thousand Oaks after riding here because Los Robles is the quintessential Santa Monica Mountains singletrack and just one of many riding options to be found in this area. Unlike the San Gabriel Mountains, the air is usually pretty clean in the Santa Monicas, and the trail traffic can be lighter, although Los Robles is pretty popular. This trail gives the rider a healthy dose of technical challenges, switchbacks, some minor rock gardens, and enough ruts and embedded rocks to keep the rider on his or her toes.

Description

The trailhead is easy to find at the northwestern end of this small parking lot. To start the ride, step over the 1-foot-high steel bar at the entrance; I've seen the disastrous results of a collision with this bar at high speed, so don't forget about if it gets dark! A large tabletop jump will quickly appear on your right as you roll the first 0.4 miles of fire road before the start of Los Robles Trail. To avoid ride-ending injuries, resist the urge to jump until the conclusion of the route and just keep spinning. There are two possible navigational mishaps in the first half mile—a right turn that you will *not* make down the Oak Creek Canyon Loop at 0.3 miles, and a fork where you'll turn right on Los Robles Trail West. Both junctions are clearly marked with signs.

The first 2 miles involve nearly 700 feet of elevation gain, but don't let that modest number fool you. This is a

GPS TRAILHEAD COORDINATES (WGS84)

UTM Zone 11S
Easting 326545
Northing 3782811
Latitude N 34.10'19"
Longitude W 118.52'54"

DIRECTIONS

From Los Angeles, take US 101 north to Thousand Oaks; exit at Moorpark Road, and turn left. Follow Moorpark Road until it ends after 0.5 miles. Park in the small dirt parking lot on the right, at the corner of Moorpark Road and Green Meadow Avenue. The trailhead is located in the northwestern end of this lot.

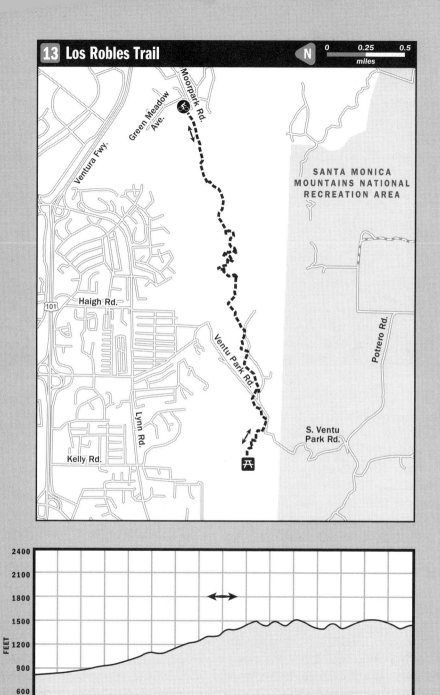

Moorpark Rd.

Green Meadow Ave.

Ventura Fwy.

SANTA MONICA
MOUNTAINS NATIONAL
RECREATION AREA

101

Haigh Rd.

Ventu Park Rd.

Potero Rd.

Lynn Rd.

S. Ventu
Park Rd.

Kelly Rd.

FEET

| 2400 |
| 2100 |
| 1800 |
| 1500 |
| 1200 |
| 900 |
| 600 |
| 300 |
| 0 |

0.89   1.79   2.68   3.58

MILES

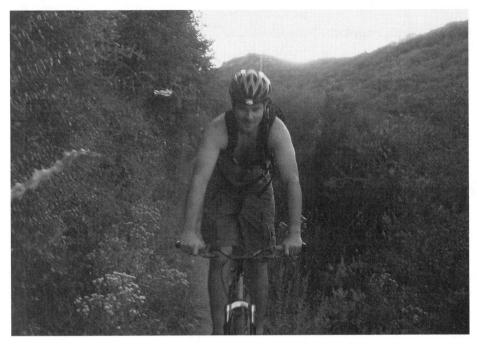

Proper summer attire on Los Robles Trail

technical climb, so you will expend a lot of extra energy negotiating switchbacks and rocky sections that will require acceleration and finesse—unlike on a fire-road climb, where you can slump back in your saddle and nearly fall asleep. Full suspension is a plus on this climb because of the embedded rocks all over the place that block your path. The author has found this climb to be much easier on a 32-pound twin-shocker than on a 22-pound XC hardtail because of the added control and forgiveness that suspension provides.

A major plus of Los Robles is the fact that the hardest part of the climb stays shaded most of the way in an otherwise blazingly hot portion of real estate. Mountain bike traffic is heavy both ways, and there are plenty of runners and dog walkers too. A forgotten relic of mountain bike evolution is quite common here—the handlebar-mounted bell—because of the busyness and numerous blind corners. If you still have one in your toolbox, dust it off and use it for this ride, although it may look out of place on your modern front end.

After the 2-mile mark, the trail starts to flatten and straighten, and there are even a few short descents before a three-way junction at just over 3 miles from the start. Avoid the downhill left turn, and continue ascending for another quarter mile until you reach the summit and a picnic table. Just before the picnic table, you'll see the entrance to Rosewood Trail, which you can schedule for another day because today is all about the famed switchbacks of Los Robles.]

The view from the picnic table is spectacular, especially after dark when the city lights glow in the valley below. At any time of day, the views of the northernmost Santa Monica

Mountains, Las Posas Hills, and Simi Peak are breathtaking and well deserving of a snap-shot or two. After telling stories and enjoying some nourishment, remount and head back down the same route you just covered.

The ride down Los Robles Trail is so much fun that you may want to lobby the park authorities to close this trail for a downhill race. Unfortunately, you cannot open up the throttle and hit peak velocity because there are other trail users around every corner—even after dark. If you have the audacity to go all out, please ride off the trail to avoid a collision with them and ensure you sustain the full brunt of physical injuries resulting from your silliness.

At the end of the ride, reward your restraint and abstinence from speed with a tweaked aerial over the large tabletop at the bottom, provided park-service officials haven't bulldozed this piece of utilitarian architecture by the time this guide is in print. Now you know why some people make the 1-hour commute to LA from Thousand Oaks and Newbury Park every morning. See a local realtor if you'd rather reserve long commutes for your professional life rather than for great mountain bike destinations like Los Robles Trail.

After the Ride

Since you just worked hard and burned many calories, you deserve a gluttonous visit to Islands Restaurant at 29271 Agoura Road in Agoura Hills; (818) 879-9933. Yes, it's a major franchise ran by a large corporation, but the burgers are world-class, and there's Newcastle Nut Brown Ale on tap.

DEAD COW/CHINA FLATS/ SUICIDE LOOP

KEY AT-A-GLANCE INFORMATION

Length: 6.5 miles

Configuration: Figure-8

Technical difficulty: 5

Aerobic difficulty: 3

Scenery: Simi Peak, Simi Hills

Exposure: 90% exposed to sunshine

Trail traffic: Light on weekdays, moderate on weekend

Trail surface: Dry hardpack with embedded sandstone boulders and small rocks—90% singletrack

Riding time: 1–2 hours

Access: Sunrise–sunset, 7 days a week

Maps: USGS 7.5-minute quad: Thousand Oaks

Special comments: Stay away from Suicide Trail if you're a novice rider.

In Brief

Just 6.5 miles long, the Dead Cow/China Flats/Suicide Loop is scarcely a test of one's aerobic capabilities on a mountain bike. It is, however, a challenging test of two-wheeled technical prowess. If you have any doubts about this particular skill set, avoid this route entirely. To complete this trail with grace, you must be a stellar technical climber and downhiller, which are two terms rarely uttered in the same breath. A dab-free day in this area is a medal of honor bestowed upon few mortals, or rather, immortals.

Description

After you've geared up, said your prayers, and strapped on knee pads and elbow guards, go around the gate at the end of King James Court and start ascending the vaunted Dead Cow singletrack.

The 1.2-mile ascent wouldn't be an easy spin if it were a groomed fire road—you gain roughly 850 feet along the way. Adding to the steepness is a minefield of embedded sandstone dab traps. The key to cleaning this climb, I've been told, is to keep up your momentum as you loft your front wheel over the rocky obstacles. As impossible as it may seem, the climb has been ridden without a dab. To do it, you've got to be on the top of your cardiovascular and technical games. Riders adept at both are few and far between because downhillers generally aren't uphill inclined, and XC specialists generally shy away from rocks. It's as if John Tomac never lived.

GPS TRAILHEAD COORDINATES (WGS84)

UTM Zone 11S
Easting 336281
Northing 3785253
Latitude N 34.11'44"
Longitude W 118.46'37"

DIRECTIONS

From Los Angeles, take US 101 northbound to Thousand Oaks and exit at Lindero Canyon Road. Turn right (north) onto Lindero Canyon, and continue for 3.8 miles; then turn left onto King James Court. After about a tenth of a mile, you'll come to a dead end where you can park. The trailhead lies at the end of King James Court.

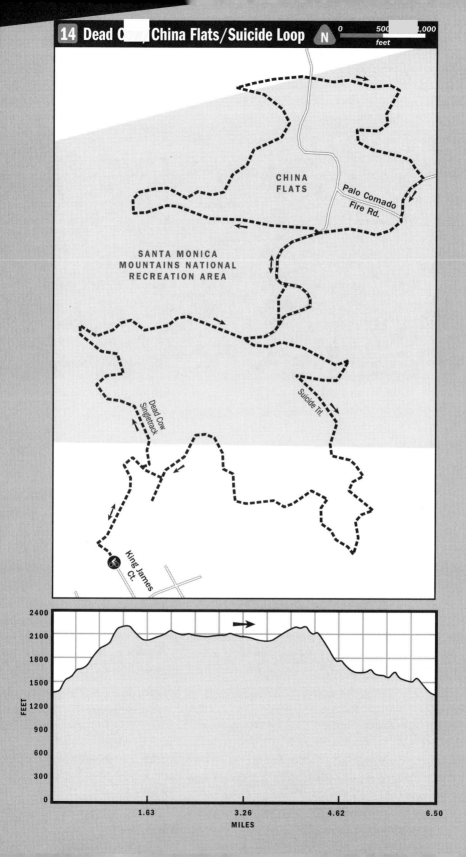

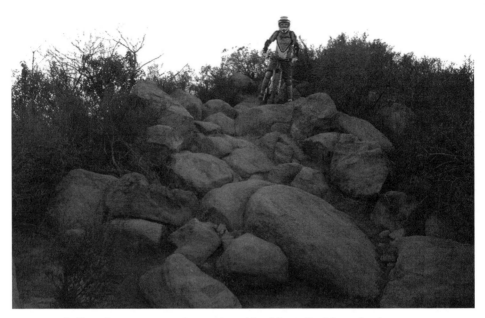

**Believe it or not, people used to ride this trail without body armor
or long-travel suspension.**

Once at the summit, you'll notice a rocky, narrow path that splits off the main trail over a small hill to your right. This is the start of Suicide Trail. Save that treat for later and continue on the main trail around a gate to the beginning of a short loop around China Flats.

After a 0.3-mile descent, veer left at the 1.6-mile mark for a short singletrack climb that ends at the 2-mile mark, after which is a fairly level, zigzagging section of trail that crosses a fire road at the 2.8-mile mark and ends at a perpendicular fire road. Turn right at the fire road, and then turn right at the 3.5-mile mark, heading west on singletrack. This little loop diversion ends roughly 3.7 miles from its start, after which a left turn will have you heading south, retracing your tire tracks back to the base of Suicide Trail.

The first few feet of Suicide are impassable on wheels, so carry your bike up the small hill. Once you get to the start of the Suicide descent, peer down at the wickedly steep and rocky chute so you can pick a safe line before you start your descent (keep your weight back as far as possible to avoid the dreaded endo). If you're in one piece at the 5.2-mile mark, turn right the first chance you get, and begin the comparatively mundane singletrack traverse back to the lower end of Dead Cow.

After the Ride

For Mexican food and margaritas to soothe the pain of injuries sustained on Suicide Trail, check out Cisco's Mexican Restaurant, at 1712 East Avenida De Los Arboles, Thousand Oaks; (805) 493-0533. For one of the area's best diners, check out Du-Par's Restaurant, at 75 West Thousand Oaks Boulevard in Thousand Oaks; (805) 373-8785.

15

KEY AT-A-GLANCE INFORMATION

Length: 9.4 miles

Configuration: Loop

Technical difficulty: 3

Aerobic difficulty: 3

Scenery: Simi Hills, Santa Monica Mountains

Exposure: 70% exposed to sunshine, shaded in Cheeseboro Canyon descent

Trail traffic: Moderate—heavy

Trail surface: Dry hardpack with some loose, rocky areas and small, sandstone slickrock formations— 30% singletrack

Riding time: 1—2 hours

Access: Sunrise—sunset, 7 days a week

Maps: USGS 7.5-minute quad: Calabasas

Special comments: Area can be extremely hot in summer, so bring plenty of water and sunblock.

GPS TRAILHEAD COORDINATES (WGS84)

UTM Zone 11S
Easting 340440
Northing 3780850
Latitude N 34.09'23"
Longitude W 118.43'51"

CHEESEBORO TO SULFUR SPRINGS LOOP

In Brief

The Cheeseboro Ridge/Sulfur Springs Loop is the perfect after-work excursion because it mixes just the right amount of technical descending, aerobic climbing, and desert and chaparral scenery into a nice, compact package. For this reason, this route is a staple of the North Valley XC scene and even entices regular visitors from other areas. Of all the rides in SoCal, Cheeseboro Ridge has the potential to be the hottest so riding this route in the late afternoon or early morning is a far better option than attacking it midday.

Description

Park your vehicle for free, carefully mount your front wheel, hit the trailhead at the northeast end of the second (larger) parking area, and head east for 0.2 miles, then head north on Cheeseboro Canyon Trail, which is actually a fire road. After 1.4 nearly level miles, leave the riparian landscape behind and turn right up the Cheeseboro Ridge Fire Road to get the blood flowing.

After 0.6 miles, turn left on Cheeseboro Ridge instead of going straight and continuing to Las Virgenes Canyon. You may start to wonder why the flora is so different here from other parts the Santa Monica Mountains. Years of cattle grazing have left the Cheeseboro Canyon area with nothing more than brush and oak trees, contrasting with the plethora of bushes, small trees, and shrubs that compose other

DIRECTIONS

From Los Angeles and the San Fernando Valley, take US 101 north and exit at Cheeseboro. Briefly head north on Palo Comado Canyon Drive; then make a right onto Cheeseboro Road. After 0.75 miles, turn right into the first parking lot, beyond which is a driveway that leads to a second, larger parking area with bathroom facilities.

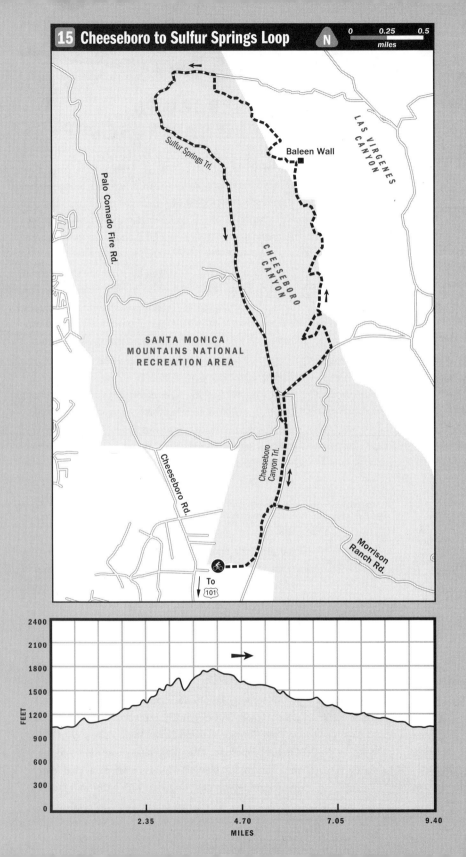

N

0   0.25   0.5
miles

Baleen Wall

LAS VIRGENES CANYON

Sulfur Springs Trl.

Palo Comado Fire Rd.

CHEESEBORO CANYON

SANTA MONICA
MOUNTAINS NATIONAL
RECREATION AREA

Cheeseboro Rd.

Cheeseboro Canyon Trl.

Morrison
Ranch Rd.

To
101

2400
2100
1800
1500
1200
900
600
300
0

FEET

2.35   4.70   7.05   9.40

MILES

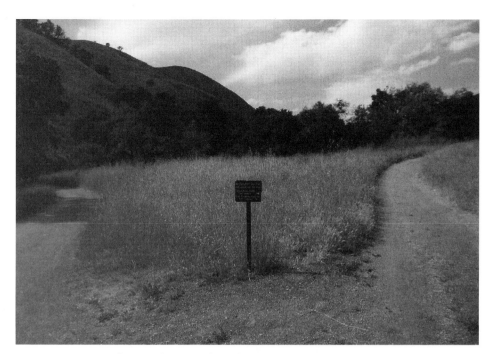

Who needs GPS when there are signs everywhere?

unmolested areas of the Santa Monicas. Livestock grazing has created millions of acres of this same landscape in the foothills of California from San Diego to the Oregon border, so you should appreciate the park service a lot more after seeing this place.

Nevertheless, this relatively new natural world has its own special beauty, despite being an entirely man-made conception. You may think the miles of grass fields would make a great habitat for snakes, and they do. If, when riding here from spring through autumn, you did not see at least one snake, you simply weren't looking hard enough. Perhaps the abundance of prey for these snakes in the grasses explains why the Cheeseboro Canyon area boasts the largest concentration of predatory birds in the lower 48.

With the exception of one really steep, loose hill, the next 1.8 miles are well-groomed fire road with no technical subtleties. The heat, however, will make you feel as if you recovered more than the measly 600-foot elevation gain over that stretch. At the 4-mile mark, you'll reach a geological formation known as the Baleen Wall—a rocky structure to perch atop while sipping H_2O and eating mountain bike confections. See if you can spot birds of prey as you peer across the vista, which includes Las Virgenes Canyon, Bell Canyon, and the Simi Hills. The land formations below provide an indication of what the area would look like without years of livestock grazing.

Two small climbs between two descents will be featured in the next 1.4 miles, with some loose rocks to keep you at attention. Stay left to avoid going up a nasty hill to the north, and after a brief bit of singletrack, turn left onto the famous Sulfur Springs Trail, roughly 5.4 miles from the start. The trail descends Cheeseboro Canyon and includes bumpy slickrock, tight turns, and intersections with Cheeseboro Creek, all of which will rattle your joints and put your bike prep to the test. About halfway down, a deft sense of smell will tell you this place was named aptly, and you may notice milky-colored water bubbling into the creek where the sulfuric stench is the thickest. This phenomenon isn't the result of a leaky septic system or runoff from a fireworks factory—it's purely natural and emanates from the bowels of the Earth.

Sadly, the singletrack ends at the 7.7-mile mark, where Sulfur Springs Trail widens, becomes a fire road, and merges with familiar territory just beyond the 8-mile mark. When you get back to your car, smile knowing that you beat the system and spent your free time in nature, rather than in front of the mind-numbing boob tube. You can quell your boredom at work the following day by daydreaming about riding the same route in reverse.

After the Ride

Since you just worked hard and burned many calories, you deserve a gluttonous visit to Islands Restaurant at 29271 Agoura Road in Agoura Hills; (818) 879-9933. Yes, it's a major franchise ran by a large corporation, but the burgers are world-class, and there's Newcastle Nut Brown Ale on tap.

16

KEY AT-A-GLANCE INFORMATION

Length: 11 miles

Configuration: Loop

Technical difficulty: 5

Aerobic difficulty: 3

Scenery: Simi Valley, Rocky Peak, Santa Monica Mountains

Exposure: 100% exposed to sunshine

Trail traffic: Moderate–heavy on weekdays, heavy on weekends

Trail surface: Hardpack with large, embedded rocks—40% single-track

Riding time: 1.5–2.5 hours

Access: Sunrise–sunset, 7 days a week

Maps: USGS 7.5-minute quad: Simi Valley East

Special comments: This ride can be very hot any day of the year—very stinking hot! Bring plenty of H$_2$O and sunblock.

GPS TRAILHEAD COORDINATES (WGS84)

UTM Zone 11S
Easting 346202
Northing 3795961
Latitude N 34.17'37"
Longitude W 118.40'16"

CHUMASH/ROCKY PEAK/ HUMMINGBIRD LOOP

In Brief

This is the crown jewel of SoCal riding—a mountain-side littered with a mosaic of sandstone boulders, some as small as VW buses and some as large as ten-story apartment buildings. The sandstone is incorporated into the riding surface of this route, creating technical subtleties that require you to be spontaneous and creative with your line-picking to avoid the dreaded "endo." Riding this route without crashing demands close attention—so proceed with caution.

Description

This is one ride that's just as enjoyable in either direction, but if you'd like to descend the famed Humming-bird Trail, park at the end of Flanagan Drive. Prepare yourself mentally for a really tough climb up Chumash Trail. Dial in your air pressures, lube your chain, set your seat up high, and begin the spin up Chumash.

You'll gain 1,300 feet of elevation over 3 miles. To climb Chumash Trail, you must have plenty of energy in reserve because the trail presents one technical obstacle after the other all the way up—be ready to stand on the cranks and loft your front wheel up and over sandstone boulders at any given moment. As you pick away at the climb, you may ponder the fun to be had descending this beast. Hold out on that temptation for another day, or at least until you reach the summit at unpaved Rocky Peak Fire Road.

DIRECTIONS

From Los Angeles, take I-405 to CA 118 West. Continue about 13 miles, and exit at Yosemite Avenue. Make a quick right onto Flanagan Drive and continue 0.8 miles until the end. Park anywhere. The clearly visible trail-head is directly at the end of Flanagan and is marked with park-service signs.

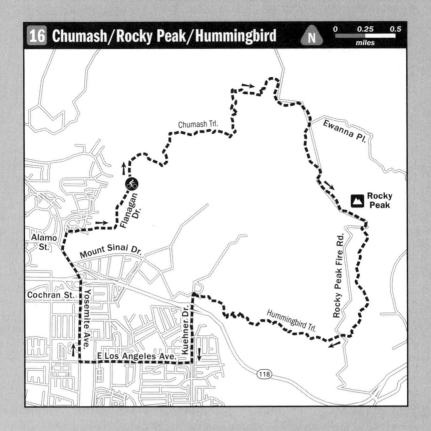

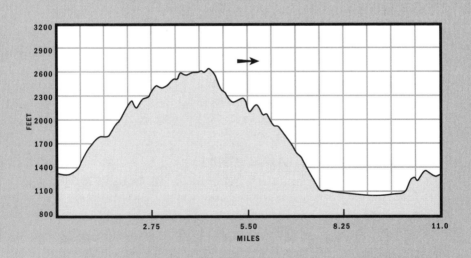

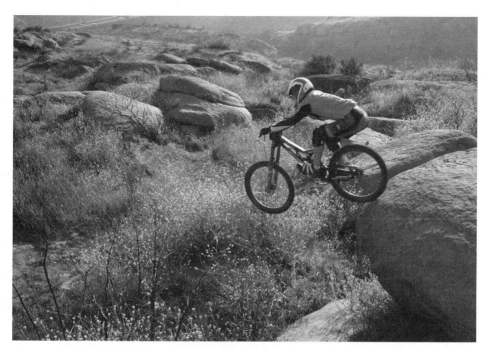

Gabriela Williams demonstrates how *not* to ride at Rocky Peak.

At the fire road, you'll turn right and spin along the west side of Rocky Peak. The first descent starts roughly 0.75 miles after the end of Chumash. Stunt riders should keep an eye out for a large jump ramp that cuts up the hillside about 0.25 miles down this descent, but make sure you scope out the landing first, of course.

Courtesy of the area's sandstone-rich geology, the remaining mile of Rocky Peak Fire Road is very bumpy, with enough obstacles to make this foray anything but mundane. Unfortunately, all fire roads aren't created equal. At about 5.9 miles from the start of your ride, turn right to descend the Hummingbird singletrack, marked with a sign and bench.

Tight switchbacks are always tough to negotiate, but Hummingbird's rocky composition means you'll also have to navigate tight turns and rocky impediments simultaneously. Stay light on the bars and easy on the front brake, looking where you want to go instead of where you don't. The technical difficulty never lets up, so you may feel a tightening in your forearm muscles by the time you reach the empty lot at the bottom of Hummingbird Trail.

At this point, either ride back up Hummingbird and do the route in reverse, or go roughly 3.5 miles on-road to get back to your car—go left on Kuehner Drive, right on Los Angeles Avenue, right on Yosemite Avenue, and right on Flanagan; then pedal to the end.

After the Ride

Fight California's oppressive SoCal food taboos by eating hearty soul food at Les Sisters Southern Kitchen at 21818 Devonshire Street in Chatsworth; (818) 998-0755. Or head to Follow Your Heart at 21825 Sherman Way for some old-school natural food; (818) 348-3240.

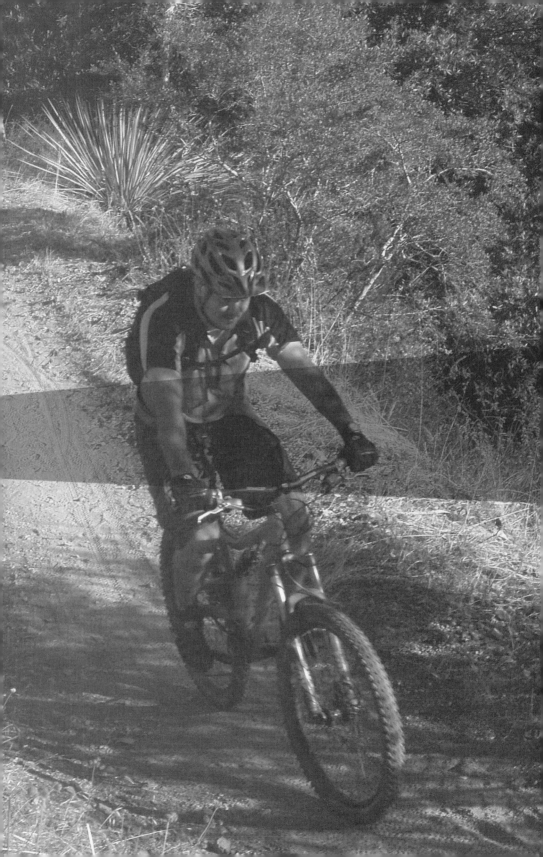

ANGELES NATIONAL FOREST

17

KEY AT-A-GLANCE INFORMATION

Length: 15.3 miles

Configuration: Figure-8

Technical difficulty: 3

Aerobic difficulty: 4

Scenery: Quail Lake, Frazier Mountain, Liebre Mountain, Antelope Valley

Exposure: 60% exposed to sunshine

Trail traffic: Very light—nonexistent

Trail surface: Varies from loam to loose and rocky surface to dry hardpack

Riding time: 2.5–3.5 hours

Access: Sunrise–sunset, 7 days a week

Maps: USGS 7.5-minute quad: Liebre Mountain

Special comments: Forest Adventure Pass is required for each vehicle parked. These can be purchased for $5 from various private vendors and ranger stations listed at **www .fs.fed.us/r5/sanbernardino/ap/ welcome.shtml.** OHVs (off-highway vehicles) are allowed in this area, so be wary of them.

GPS TRAILHEAD COORDINATES (WGS84)

UTM Zone   11S
Easting   343694
Northing   3845413
Latitude   N 34.44'20"
Longitude   W 118.42'27"

LIEBRE MOUNTAIN/ GOLDEN EAGLE TRAIL

In Brief

Treasured by the few who know about this route, the Liebre Mountain/Golden Eagle Trail is one of the best rides accessible from Los Angeles. The narrow single-track descent is an idyllic, seemingly perfect stretch that differs from other SoCal trails in that it lacks steepness and rocky imperfections. Momentum can be acquired only by pedaling, but you want to take it slow and soak in the heavenly natural splendor all around. The trail is such a gem that you may not believe it's open to and regularly used by off-road motorcyclists, as well as hikers, horseback riders, and cyclists. Golden Eagle Trail is living proof that public lands aren't destroyed when used for a variety of recreational pursuits, despite the opinions of foot-traffic-only advocates.

Description

Since you probably won't encounter another rider on the trail, pack all the tools, tubes, and patch kits you need to be fully self-sufficient. Start riding south on the Old Ridge Route. This was the only way to transgress the mountains in this area way back in 1915 when the road was built. Along the way, you may notice exposed bits of the granite cobblestone that formed the old road's foundation.

After about 2.75 miles of mild descending, turn left at the first opportunity, onto a dirt road marked 7N23. The

DIRECTIONS

From Los Angeles, take Interstate 405 northbound toward Sacramento until it becomes I-5. Stay on I-5 north about 39 miles until you reach the exit for CA 138 east toward Lancaster–Palmdale. After about 2.5 miles, turn right onto the Old Ridge Route; continue on the Old Ridge Route about 2.7 miles until you reach the small town of Sandberg, California. Park your car with your Forest Adventure Pass displayed.

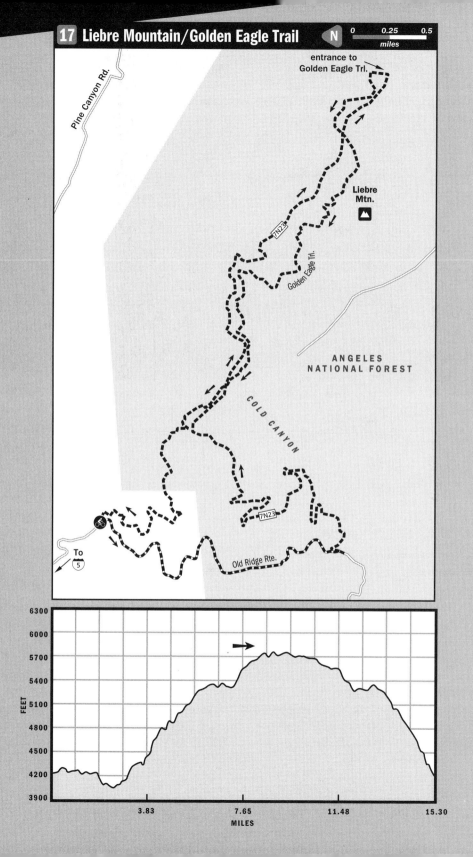

entrance to
Golden Eagle Trl.

Pine Canyon Rd.

Liebre
Mtn.

7N23

Golden Eagle Trl.

ANGELES
NATIONAL FOREST

COLD CANYON

7N23

Old Ridge Rte.

To
5

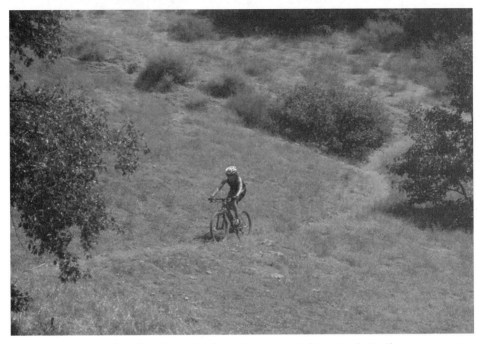

Maria Biber-Ferro far from home on Golden Eagle Trail

toughest climbing of the day occurs within the first 4 miles on this road—you'll gain more than 1,300 feet of elevation. If you get really lucky, you'll see the bird of prey whose name the trail you'll later descend bears. If you look down at the ground, you'll need even less luck to spot the California horned lizard, which is very common to this area. Clear skies are all you need for the great views, including but not limited to Cold Canyon, Liebre Mountain, Bald Mountain, the Tehachapi Mountains, and all the unnamed peaks, hills, and valleys of the Angeles National Forest.

At 9.25 miles, after nearly 1,800 feet of elevation gain, the climbing will end as you turn left to begin the Golden Eagle Trail descent. If you came for an adrenaline rush, you won't find it here—this singletrack is laid-back and mellow. If you want speed, you'll have to earn it with pedal strokes. The trail crosses the road at the 10-mile mark, then again after roughly 12.9 miles from the start, after which it gets significantly steeper and keeps you on a fast but untechnical clip until it ends and rejoins with Old Ridge Road and takes you to your car, about 15.3 miles from the start.

After the Ride

Dining options are virtually nil in the Liebre Mountain area, so bring your own nutritious spread in a cooler for instant postride refreshment.

18

FIVE DEER TRAIL

KEY AT-A-GLANCE INFORMATION

Length: 11 miles

Configuration: Loop

Technical difficulty: 3

Aerobic difficulty: 3

Scenery: Bouquet Reservoir, Bouquet Canyon, Martindale Canyon, Sierra Pelona Mountains, Sleepy Valley

Exposure: 70% exposed to sunshine

Trail traffic: Light–moderate on weekdays, moderate on weekends

Trail surface: Dry hardpack with embedded and loose rocks

Riding time: 1.5–2.5 hours

Access: Sunrise–sunset, 7 days a week

Maps: USGS 7.5-minute quad: Sleepy Valley

Special comments: A Forest Adventure Pass must be purchased for each vehicle parked. These can be purchased for $5 from various private vendors and ranger stations listed at **www.fs.fed.us/r5/san bernardino/ap/welcome.shtml.**

GPS TRAILHEAD COORDINATES (WGS84)

UTM Zone   11S

Easting   374802

Northing   3827391

Latitude   N 34.34'50"

Longitude   W 118.21'54"

In Brief

The Five Deer Trail is a surprisingly pristine single-track within the highly popular off-highway-vehicle (OHV) area called Rowher Flats. Although there are many great trails located within OHV areas in SoCal, none have lighter OHV traffic than Five Deer Trail because of its elusive location and sliver width. Even if you do find yourself dodging a few dirt bikes, you'd be hard-pressed to find a better piece of singletrack anywhere in the vicinity of LA County.

Description

Park your rig, hang your Forest Adventure Pass, hop on your cycle, and start spinning east on Forest Service Road 6N08. Like most service roads, the elevation gain is steady and mellow. As you rise up the road, lots of great scenery will come into view—the Bouquet Reservoir, Jupiter Mountain, Martindale Canyon, and Leona Valley, to name a few. Relax and enjoy the leisurely 4.8-mile climb with a paltry 1,500-foot elevation gain.

DIRECTIONS

From Los Angeles, take I-405 northbound toward Sacramento, and then converge with I-5 northbound. Continue on I-5 about 3 miles, merge with CA 14 north toward Lancaster-Palmdale 8.5 miles, and exit CA 14 at Sand Canyon Road. Turn left and drive on Sand Canyon Road about 2 miles until you reach Sierra Highway; go right. Stay on Sierra Highway about 0.4 miles, and then turn left onto Vasquez Canyon Road. Continue on Vasquez about 3.5 miles until you reach Bouquet Canyon Road; then turn right. After roughly 9.7 miles on Bouquet Canyon Road, look for the Bouquet Canyon Dam and the Bouquet Canyon Reservoir. About 1 mile beyond where the road passes the dam on your left, turn right onto a dirt road marked 6N08. About 0.5 miles up this dirt road, another dirt road, marked 6N06, intersects it. Park at the intersection, being sure to display your Forest Adventure Pass.

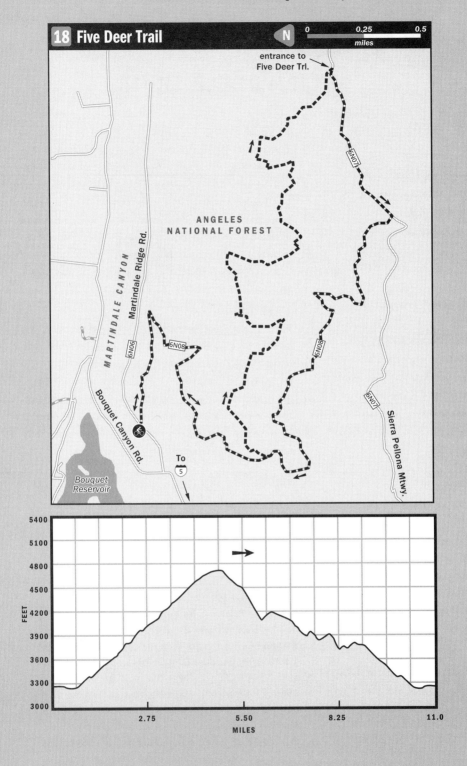

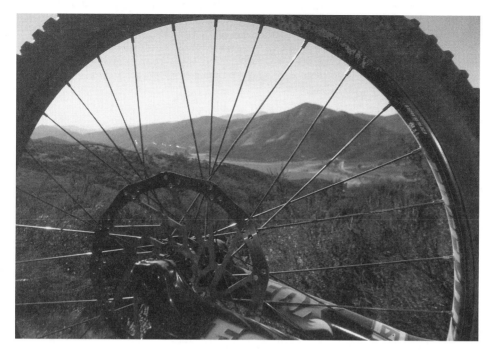

Vista behind mountain bike wheel

You won't find any navigational mishaps on your way to the summit; just stay on the wide, groomed road and avoid the rutty, steep Jeep road that periodically intersects it. At the 4.4-mile mark, sit down and enjoy another majestic panorama of the surrounding mountains and valleys, including Mount McDill, Sierra Pelona Valley, and Soledad Canyon.

After your break, cross over the fence and start descending FS 6N07, which is easy to spot because it's the only option available. Look for the entrance to Five Deer Trail, which is on the left side of FS 6N07, about 0.9 miles from the cancellation of FS 6N08, and roughly 5.3 miles from the start of the route. It's the only singletrack that descends to the west.

The first mile of Five Deer Trail is very steep and marred with deep ruts that present a technical challenge. To avoid mishap, repeat these words to yourself over and over: "Look where I want to go, not where I don't want to go." Sounds silly, but it works. For some reason, the hands respond involuntarily to visual input. You will turn where you look; remember that.

The grade mellows out shortly, and Five Deer becomes what you came for—a snaking, narrow, peaceful, pristine singletrack not unlike the trails pictured in every mountain bike mag. You can thank the dirt bikers for keeping this trail passable. Without their visits, the trail would be so overgrown that you'd have to crawl through almost impenetrably dense foliage on your hands and knees.

After crossing a few Jeep roads, you'll sadly find the singletrack comes to an end at the 9-mile mark, after which you'll turn right and retrace your tracks to your vehicle. If you have a dirt bike, come back another day and give Five Deer a shot using petrol instead of carbohydrates—and do it quick, because dirt bikes are very close to being outlawed on all public lands in California.

19

CHILAO FLAT: MOUNT HILLYER LOOP

KEY AT-A-GLANCE INFORMATION

Length: 8.7 miles

Configuration: Loop with 1.2-mile spur

Technical difficulty: 4

Aerobic difficulty: 3

Scenery: Broad panorama of San Gabriel Mountains atop Mt. Hillyer

Exposure: 50% exposed

Trail traffic: Light on weekends and weekdays

Trail surface: Pine-needle loam, loose granite rocks, sand—40% singletrack

Riding time: 2–3 hours

Access: Sunrise–sunset, 7 days a week

Maps: USGS 7.5-minute quad: Chilao Flat

Special comments: This area can be very hot in summer and cold enough for snowfall during winter, so prepare accordingly. Forest Adventure Passes are required for all vehicles parked here. These can be purchased for $5 from various private vendors and ranger stations listed at www.fs.fed.us/r5/san bernardino/ap/welcome.shtml.

GPS TRAILHEAD COORDINATES (WGS84)

UTM Zone   11S
Easting   406892
Northing   3799328
Latitude   N 34.19'52"
Longitude W 118.00'44"

In Brief

The Chilao Flat area provides a mountain bike experience that is vastly different from that of the other routes in the San Gabriel Mountains. Instead of 2,000-plus-foot climbs and steep, vertigo-inspiring descents, the Chilao area provides two separate loops that, although aerobically challenging, are characterized by mild climbs and descents through a hilly rather than mountainous pine forest. Deep in the heart of the Angeles National Forest, the Mount Hillyer Loop is more technical than its mellower sibling—the Vetter Mountain Loop, which is also covered in this book. Perhaps the perfect time to enjoy this route would be before or after a mild snowstorm in the winter. Just make sure you bring your all-wheel-drive vehicle.

Description

Once you've parked your vehicle near the intersection of Silver Moccasin Trail and Forest Service Road 3N21 (the road that passes the Chilao Visitor Center), hop on your steed and pedal west on FS 3N21 just over 0.3 miles, and turn right on FS 3N14.

The pavement ends at roughly the 1.4-mile mark. The ride continues with a mild ascent toward Alder Saddle that features majestic views of the Granite and Pacifico Mountains to your left. Turn right onto the dirt road marked FS 3N17, which becomes pavement and descends for a mile. At about the 4.35-mile mark, turn right onto

DIRECTIONS

From I-210 in La Cañada, drive on the Angeles Crest Highway (CA 2) about 25 miles. Just beyond the Chilao Campground is the Chilao Visitor Center, which is clearly marked with a sign on your left side. Turn left into this driveway, and park near the entrance to Silver Moccasin Trail, which is about 0.5 miles beyond the visitor center. Don't forget to hang your Forest Adventure Pass from the rearview mirror.

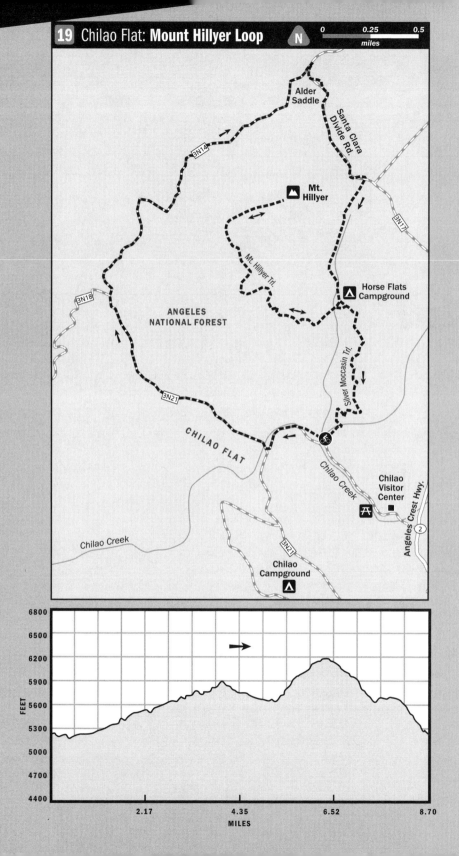

19 Chilao Flat: **Mount Hillyer Loop**

N

0   0.25   0.5
miles

Alder
Saddle

Santa Clara
Divide Rd.

3N14

Mt.
Hillyer

3N17

Mt. Hillyer Trl.

Horse Flats
Campground

3N18

ANGELES
NATIONAL FOREST

Silver Moccasin Trl.

3N21

CHILAO FLAT

Chilao Creek

Chilao
Visitor
Center

Angeles Crest Hwy.

2

Chilao Creek

3N21

Chilao
Campground

FEET

6800
6500
6200
5900
5600
5300
5000
4700
4400

2.17   4.35   6.52   8.70

MILES

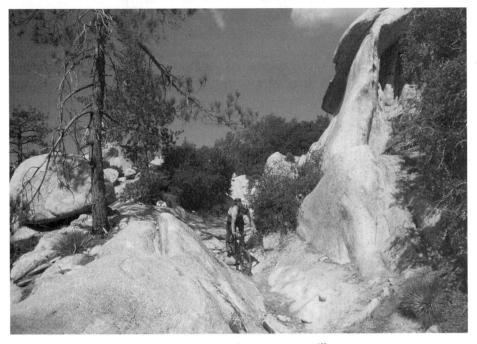

Rubber meets granite at Mount Hillyer.

the road that leads you to Horse Flats Campground, where both Mount Hillyer and Silver Moccasin trails begin.

For the most technical riding of the day, head southwest, ascending Mount Hillyer Trail. It's a sketchy stretch, so you'll definitely be walking or carrying your bike over more than a few obstacles. Just think of what fun they'll be on the way down, and keep going. At roughly the 6.4-mile mark, you'll reach the summit of Mount Hillyer, where you can enjoy 360-degree views of the natural splendor that is Angeles National Forest. You can also be thankful that Mount Hillyer is outside the San Gabriel Wilderness boundaries, within which, due to the efforts of foot-traffic-only advocates, bike travel is forbidden.

The Mount Hillyer Trail descent is a hoot that begs to be ridden over and over again. You can choose from multiple lines, plus several air-catching opportunities along the way. Although Mount Hillyer Trail ends at roughly the 7.6-mile mark, the fun doesn't, because now you get to descend Silver Moccasin Trail back to your car.

Silver Moccasin's technical challenges come in the form of man-made obstacles rather than natural subtleties. Several log steps form one- to two-foot drops all the way down. If you choose to roll over these steps, get your weight as far back as possible, or loft your front wheel and "wheelie drop" it—but do so with adequate speed, or you may crash.

At 8.8 miles, you're at the end of the more technical sibling of the two loops at Chilao Flat. Bring a wholesome spread of food and cold beverages to replenish your energy for the Vetter Mountain Loop (see next profile), which will make it an epic day. Shoot, any day spent riding your bike is good day, so don't feel bad if you can't muster the zeal to ride any longer—you're out of the rat race, and that's good enough.

CHILAO FLAT:
VETTER MOUNTAIN LOOP

KEY AT-A-GLANCE INFORMATION

Length: 12 miles

Configuration: Loop

Technical difficulty: 3

Aerobic difficulty: 3

Scenery: All-encompassing panorama of San Gabriel Mountains from Vetter Mountain fire lookout

Exposure: 60% exposed to sunshine

Trail traffic: Always light

Trail surface: Loam, loose granite rocks, sand—38% singletrack

Riding time: 2–3 hours

Access: Sunrise–sunset, 7 days a week

Maps: USGS 7.5-minute quads: Chilao Flat, Waterman Mountain

Special comments: This area can be very hot in summer and cold enough for snowfall during winter, so prepare accordingly. Forest Adventure Passes are required for all vehicles parking here. These can be purchased for $5 from various private vendors and ranger stations listed at **www.fs.fed.us/r5/sanbernardino/ap/welcome.shtml.**

GPS TRAILHEAD COORDINATES (WGS84)
UTM Zone 11S
Easting 406905
Northing 3799355
Latitude N 34.19'53"
Longitude W 118.00'43"

In Brief

More aerobically challenging than its previously profiled sister ride, the Vetter Mountain Loop provides an adventure uncharacteristic of the other routes in the San Gabriel Mountains area, lacking sweat-drenching, painful 3,000-foot uphill grinds and dangerous, cliff-edged, narrow-switchback descents. Instead, the Vetter Mountain Loop offers a laid-back, up-and-down trot that stays within 1,000 feet of its starting elevation the whole way, and any spill will result in dirty clothing rather than untimely death.

Description

Start on the Silver Moccasin Trail, pedaling south. This trail is pure bliss—a loamy, forest-floor, tire-width gem that meanders up and down, snaking through the trees. The brief steep climb that ends at the 0.6-mile mark is the last bit of masochism you'll experience, but you'll get a workout in the miles ahead.

After a short descent, cross Forest Service Road 3N21 at roughly the 0.9-mile mark, continue uphill, and follow with a fast descent that ends at the 1.75-mile mark, at which you'll turn left at a junction. The singletrack ends at the 2.8-mile mark, where you'll turn right onto paved FS 3N16. This ascent takes you through the Charlton Flats Campground and ends at a T-junction at roughly the 4.25-mile mark, where you'll turn right to start the ascent to Vetter Mountain.

DIRECTIONS

From I-210 in La Cañada, drive on the Angeles Crest Highway (CA 2) about 25 miles. Just beyond the Chilao Campground is the Chilao Visitor Center, which is clearly marked with a sign on your left side. Turn left into this driveway, and park near the entrance to Silver Moccasin Trail, which is about 0.5 miles beyond the visitor center. Don't forget to hang your Forest Adventure Pass from the rearview mirror.

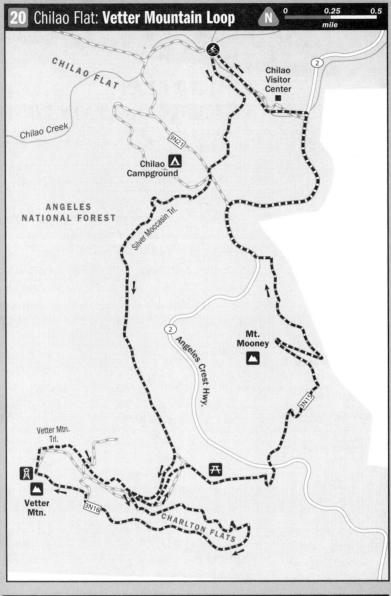

N

0	0.25	0.5

mile

CHILAO FLAT

Chilao Creek

Chilao
Visitor
Center

2

3N21

Chilao
Campground

ANGELES
NATIONAL FOREST

Silver Moccasin Trl.

2

Angeles Crest Hwy.

Mt.
Mooney

3N15

Vetter Mtn.
Trl.

Vetter
Mtn.

3N16

CHARLTON FLATS

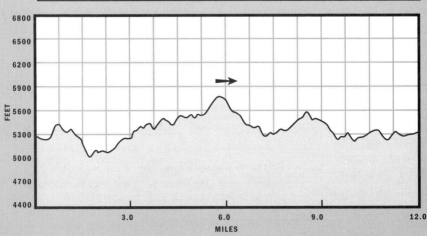

FEET

MILES

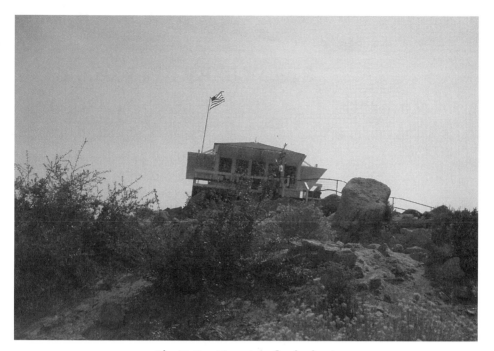

The Vetter Mountain fire lookout

The road turns to dirt and steeper in the last half mile, ending at the 5.8-mile mark. Perched atop Vetter Mountain is a fully functioning fire lookout, one of the last of its kind in California. If you show up on the right day, a volunteer firefighter will be there to welcome you and give you a tour. The lookout is appropriately placed: Vetter Mountain has a 360-degree view of the surrounding mountains and forest. Drop a buck or two in the donation box before you head down to the picnic table for a snack.

Right down the hill below the picnic table is the entrance to Vetter Mountain Trail, which is signposted. The descent is tight, slightly overgrown, and deeply rutted, but no disastrous consequences loom. You'll cross a road at the 6.5-mile mark. Continue down the increasingly fun trail, and make another, more-familiar road crossing at about the 6.8-mile mark. The remaining 0.4-mile stretch parallels the stretch of FS 3N16 you crossed earlier.

Vetter Mountain Trail ends at the 7.3-mile mark, where you'll turn right and cross the familiar territory of the Charlton Flats Campground; turn left to head back to CA 2, the Angeles Crest Highway. Since pavement is boring, turn right onto the first road that comes into view (FS 3N15) after briefly heading west on CA 2, and begin the easy ascent to Mount Mooney. After about 8.6 miles, crest the top of Mount Mooney, turn left, and bomb back down to CA 2, where you'll turn right to begin a 2-mile spin back to Chilao Visitor Center and your car.

If you're ready for more action, refuel at your car and embark on the Mount Hillyer Loop for a less aerobic but more technically challenging ride. Or relax and savor the idyllic alpine environment of Chilao Flat, pondering when you'll be able to come back and experience it all over again.

STRAWBERRY PEAK LOOP

Length: 14.8 miles

Configuration: Loop

Technical difficulty: 4

Aerobic difficulty: 4

Scenery: Strawberry Peak, Josephine Peak, Mount Lawlor, San Gabriel Mountains

Exposure: 50% exposed to sun

Trail traffic: Light on weekdays, light to moderate on weekends

Trail surface: Mostly loose and rocky, with some sandy and loamy sections—95% singletrack

Riding time: 2.5–3.5 hours

Access: Sunrise–sunset, 7 days

Maps: USGS 7.5-minute topo: Condor Peak, Chilao Flat

Special comments: To park your vehicle in this area, you must display a Forest Adventure Pass on your car. These can be purchased for $5 from various private vendors and ranger stations listed at **www .fs.fed.us/r5/sanbernardino/ap/ welcome.shtml.**

GPS TRAILHEAD COORDINATES (WGS84)

UTM Zone   11S
Easting   393883
Northing   3792738
Latitude   N 34.16'16"
Longitude   W 118.09'12"

In Brief

The Strawberry Peak Loop is another reason the San Gabriel Mountains rank as the premier mountain bike destination in Southern California. Although it's very sketchy, this route doesn't get top honors in the technical department, but it is without a doubt the scariest. Can you handle riding on the edge of a cliff for extended periods? If you're affected by vertigo, then ride somewhere else— *anywhere else*—because you won't find a more exposed ride in the southern half of the Golden State. It is also one of the best singletrack experiences to be had anywhere, and surely one to write home about.

Safety Message

Because of the trail's technical difficulty and nearness to disastrous drop-offs and cliffs, no novice riders should attempt this ride under any circumstances. *Never* attempt this route alone or late in the day.

Description

The underlying philosophy behind the design of the routes in this book is to save the technical riding for the descent rather than the climb. After all, we're not riding unsuspended rigid mountain bikes, looking for the smoothest way down the hill. So park your car at the top

DIRECTIONS

From Los Angeles, take I-110 north toward Pasadena until you reach the I-5 exit; head north on I-5 1.9 miles toward Sacramento, then head north on CA 2 toward Glendale about 7.6 miles, then take I-210 east toward Pasadena briefly, and, finally, go north on CA 2, the Angeles Crest Highway, about 9.7 miles. Keep an eye out for Switzer Picnic Area, and park in the lot at the top of the driveway that heads down to it. Don't forget to hang a Forest Adventure Pass from your rearview mirror.

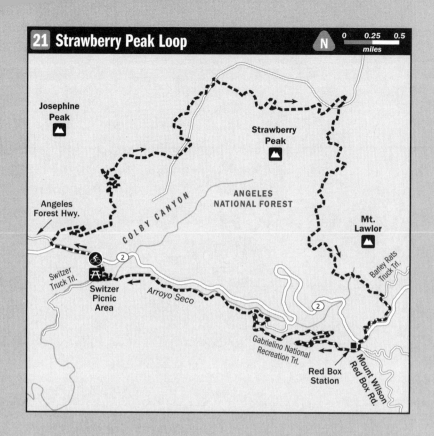

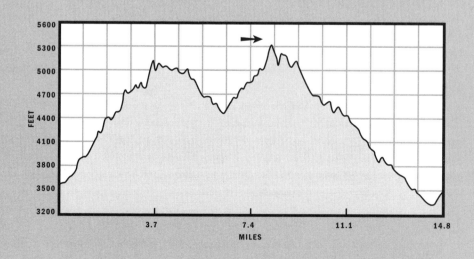

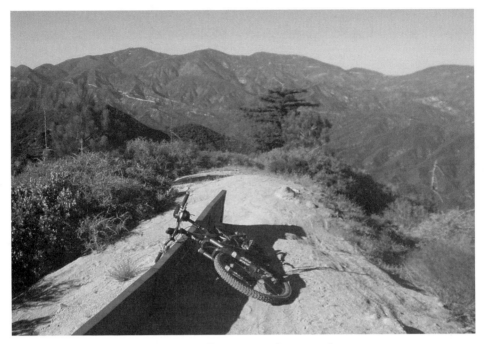

Taking it all in at Strawberry Peak

of the Switzer Picnic Area driveway, mount up, and ride your rig west about 0.4 miles; then turn right onto Angeles Forest Highway and hang another right onto the first dirt road that comes into view, about 400 feet along.

Although on paper the climb to Josephine Peak seems like a lung burner, it's the mellowest 3-mile, 1,350-foot climb to be found anywhere. The fire road never gets really steep, and its smoothness allows the rider to easily reach a meditative state in the saddle. Before you know it, you'll be crossing Josephine Saddle, which is the ridge that connects Josephine Peak to Strawberry Peak. Now you're riding singletrack, and you won't see another fire road for the rest of the day.

After roughly 3.4 miles, you'll see the turnoff for Colby Canyon Trail. Stay left and save that adventure for another day. For roughly the next 1.7 miles, the trail skirts the north side of Strawberry Peak. This part of the ride is the scariest because much of the trail is constructed on what would be rockslides. Take a minute to appreciate the efforts of whoever built and maintains this trail. The wood reinforcement is there for a reason—without it, the trail would slide down the hill—just like you will if you get too cute with your front tire. Don't fall in this section. If you do, you may not die, but you are assured at least one night's stay in the boondocks with plenty of scrapes and lacerations to keep a nice aroma of blood in the air.

The farther you go on Strawberry Peak Trail, the fewer reminders you will see of the fact that you are very close to the urban metropolis of Los Angeles. You may as well be in the Swiss Alps or the Andes Mountains, because you are in an alpine environment with no sign of civilization in sight. At roughly 5.2 miles from the start, a dandy descent will start, finishing about 6.3 miles down the trail; plenty of hunks of granite and sharp, steep turns along the way will keep you on your toes.

A navigational mishap to avoid: turning left at the trail junction at about 6.35 miles from the start. *Don't do this*—your objective is to go around Strawberry Peak clockwise. Go right and start the 1.75-mile-or-so climb to the next trail junction at the base of Mount Lawlor. Once you pass this and start your descent of Strawberry Peak Trail to the Red Box Station, you should be pretty bushed because your legs have taken you up more than 3,000 feet. Don't worry; it's basically all downhill from this point, but keep your fingers on the brake levers! Just around every corner on Strawberry Peak Trail lies a potential disaster.

After jumping the water bars on your approach to the Angeles Crest Highway, hang a right onto CA 2, make an immediate left onto Mount Wilson Road, and quickly turn right into the parking lot of Red Box Station. Follow the signs in the west end of the parking lot to the Gabrielino National Recreation Trail (NRT). The next 4.2 miles of this route are used more than Strawberry Peak Trail is, so the trail is wider. You may be relieved that you can lay off the brakes for a little while and let it all hang out, but that feeling will be short-lived. The *Yucca whipplei,* or chaparral yucca, with daggerlike leaves around its base, will keep you from getting imprecise with your steering, as will fear of making one of many disastrous cliffside meanderings. Roughly 2 miles down the Gabrielino National Recreation Trail, rock gardens will test your technical abilities and the structural integrity of your wrist bones if you choose to endo like I did.

The ride ends at the Switzer Picnic Area, where you can have your own feast, if you were so daring as to park your mobile vittle-carrier beyond the gates that close at dusk. If you were smart enough to park your car at the top of the driveway, you can have a tailgate party up there and recollect the day's action and mishaps on one of the greatest trails anywhere.

After the Ride

Beer aficionados and the malnourished should pay a visit to The Stuffed Sandwich at 1145 East Las Tunas Drive in nearby San Gabriel; (626) 285-9161. For those with a larger appetite, try Zeke's Smokehouse BBQ at 2209 Honolulu Avenue in Montrose; it has a casual atmosphere and serves ridiculously tasty cuisine that will thoroughly alleviate your carbohydrate, protein, and fat deficiencies; (818) 206-8947.

RED BOX/GABRIELINO NATIONAL RECREATION TRAIL

KEY AT-A-GLANCE INFORMATION

Length: 13.9 miles

Configuration: One-way shuttle descent

Technical difficulty: 5

Aerobic difficulty: 3

Scenery: Brown Mountain, San Gabriel Peak, Arroyo Seco Creek, numerous waterfalls

Exposure: 80% shaded by tall trees in canyon

Trail traffic: Heavy in the last few miles, light to moderate everywhere else

Trail surface: Surface composition varies greatly; including rocks, hardpack, and sand—100% singletrack

Riding time: 3–5 hours

Access: Sunrise–sunset, 7 days a week

Maps: USGS 7.5-minute quads: Pasadena, Condor Peak, Chilao Flat

In Brief

The Red Box/Gabrielino National Recreation Trail (NRT) offers the most dynamic and encompassing terrain of any one ride in Southern California. The first 6 miles is a pristine high-desert snake run with plenty of granite boulders, spiny yucca plants, and hundred-plus-foot cliffs to fall off. The middle of the ride is unlike any other in this area—a loamy, tire-width sliver of a trail that runs along moss- and fern-covered rocks, reminding you of the landscape in the *Lord of the Rings* trilogy. The end of the route is a foot-soaking hike-a-bike that will take you back to the roots of the sport. This 13.9-mile ride includes a total of 5,300 feet of descending, making it the longest continuous descent south in the Eastern Sierras' Lower Rock Creek.

Safety Message

This ride poses many dangers, and injuries can happen, so bring ample H_2O, first-aid supplies, extra layers of clothing, and a cell phone.

Description

Purists may want to ascend the Mount Wilson Toll Road to make this ride an epic all-day loop instead of a shuttle run. Unlike other shuttle runs, this route includes roughly 1,900 feet of elevation gain, courtesy of several short climbs, so shuttling to the top is by no means a lazy option. Shuttling is also advantageous because it saves

GPS TRAILHEAD COORDINATES (WGS84)

UTM Zone 11S
Easting 398209
Northing 3791349
Latitude N 34.15'30"
Longitude W 118.06'20"

DIRECTIONS

From I-210, take the Arroyo Windsor exit and head north 0.8 miles; park in the large lot on your left. The entrance to the park lies just north of this lot at the end of Windsor Drive.

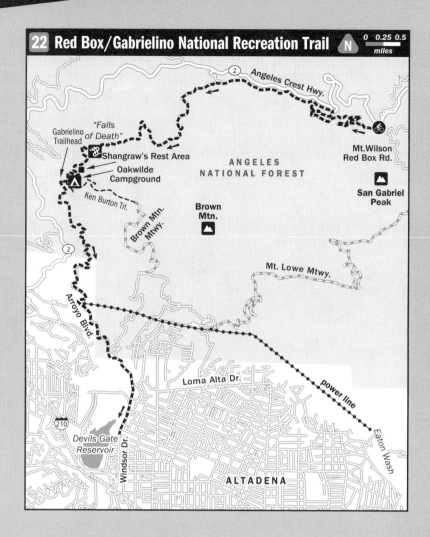

N

0   0.25 0.5
miles

Angeles Crest Hwy.

Gabrielino
Trailhead
"Falls
of Death"
Shangraw's Rest Area
Oakwilde
Campground
Ken Burton Trl.

Brown Mtn. Mtwy.

Brown
Mtn.

ANGELES
NATIONAL FOREST

Mt. Wilson
Red Box Rd.

San Gabriel
Peak

Mt. Lowe Mtwy.

Arroyo Blvd.

power line

Loma Alta Dr.

Devils Gate
Reservoir

Windsor Dr.

ALTADENA

Eaton Wash

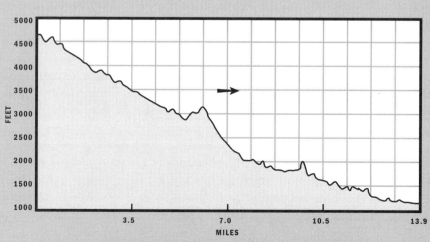

FEET

5000
4500
4000
3500
3000
2500
2000
1500
1000

3.5   7.0   10.5   13.9
MILES

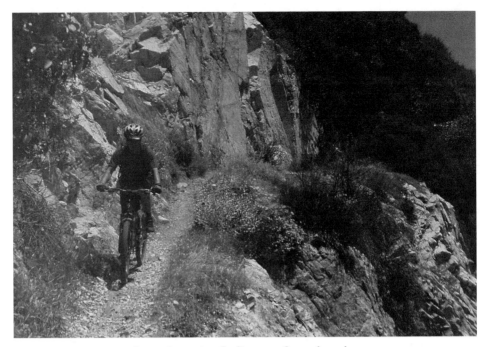

Always keep a safe distance from the edge.

your energy for the technically demanding descent and allows you to use a downhill or free-ride bike, which would be too heavy and inefficient for ascending Mount Wilson.

Once you've found the parking lot at the intersection of Mount Wilson Road and the Angeles Crest Highway, make sure your hydration pack includes the following before you start the descent: two extra tubes, tire levers, a tire pump or CO_2, a patch kit, a multitool, a chain tool with a short length of chain and extra pins, a first-aid kit, a cell phone, and some nutrition bars or snacks. These things are necessary on any ride, but they are absolutely crucial for this adventure because the Gabrielino NRT takes you far away from help, and hazards are everywhere. Novice riders should avoid this trail altogether because of its technical difficulty.

The descent starts wide and somewhat groomed, but it isn't easy, because the football-sized granite rocks strewn everywhere will deflect your front wheel over and over. After about 2.5 miles, the trail is no longer groomed, and rock gardens start appearing. These rocky sections provide a challenge, but all riders should think twice about doing them because this is only the beginning of the ride, and it is a long way out in case of a season-ending injury.

After the rock gardens, the trail meanders along a cliff. Although fencing shields the more-perilous drops, the Grim Reaper is still waiting in a number of places to pay a careless rider an early visit. Mother Nature isn't finished throwing danger at you there—she has created another hazard in the form of *Yucca whipplei,* or chaparral yucca. The bush that forms the base of this floral wonder is a bouquet of daggers that grow unusually large (up to

8 feet in diameter) in this area, and it can easily pierce a careless rider's legs. If you want to avoid massive blood loss, dismount and walk around these unmistakable obstacles.

Once you've learned to negotiate these hazards, you can enjoy this high-altitude terrain, which differs hugely from that of the Santa Monicas. The trail is far looser and composed of largely marble-sized pieces of granite rather than packed clay. In this area, granite usually indicates higher altitude, while sandstone indicates lower altitude. But as you descend into the canyon, the terrain slowly morphs to chaparral once again. Things stay familiar only briefly, however.

At roughly mile 6, the natural splendor carved out by Arroyo Seco Creek over multiple millennia dominates the trail. This strange, dark world is a virtual greenhouse, with tall trees trapping moisture and creating a fern-, moss-, and loam-draped landscape more commonly seen in the forests of the Pacific Northwest. This extremely narrow stretch of trail, which I call "Vertigo," presents the ever-present danger of falling 50-plus feet into the shallow creek below. At times, you'll find yourself stopping and staring in awe at the perfectly constructed trail ahead of you and wondering how this sanctuary eluded you in years past. Perhaps you wonder why the sign in the parking lot doesn't read "The Greatest Trail in the Milky Way Galaxy." Although the trail is narrow, traction is always ample on loam because of its moistness and lack of rocks, so you can ride this section gracefully if you focus on where you want to go instead of looking down at the certain doom to your right.

At roughly 7.5 miles from your start, you will come to another site, which I've nicknamed "The Falls of Death." A pool of water at the top of this waterfall would be great for skinny-dipping if not for the fact that its slippery walls would leave a swimmer hopelessly trapped. Death also looms for anyone who gets too intimate with the edge: the falls drop about 100 feet to a pool below. If you're wearing bike shoes with slippery cleats, stand back.

Approximately 0.5 miles beyond the falls lies Shangraw's Rest Area, which includes a single picnic table and serves as a great place to recollect your day and reflect on the adventure. Continue another half mile and pass the lower entrance to the Ken Burton Trail, just beyond which you will find the Oakwilde Campground. For people who disdain the hike-a-bike, or for pure adrenaline seekers, this parking lot is the perfect place to stage a second vehicle. The rest of the Gabrielino NRT flattens out and includes many creek crossings, impassable sand, and boulder-strewn hiking sections, so for continuous riding, avoid it and do the first 8 miles over again before sunset.

The hardier or more adventurous can head on and be rewarded with more-pristine singletrack and mesmerizing views of Arroyo Seco Creek. When you finish, you'll be dirty and sporting a few minor abrasions—very hard-core indeed.

After the Ride

For beer aficionados and the malnourished, pay a visit to The Stuffed Sandwich at 1145 East Las Tunas Drive in nearby San Gabriel; (626) 285-9161. For a larger appetite, try Zeke's Smokehouse BBQ at 2209 Honolulu Avenue in Montrose; (818) 206-8947. It has a casual atmosphere and serves ridiculously tasty cuisine that will thoroughly alleviate your carbohydrate, protein, and fat deficiencies.

KEY AT-A-GLANCE INFORMATION

Length: 15 miles

Configuration: Loop

Aerobic difficulty: 4

Technical difficulty: 4

Scenery: Massive vistas of steep, jagged peaks; deep canyons of the San Gabriels; views of Los Angeles

Exposure: No shade on Brown Mountain Road or Ken Burton singletrack; shade on Gabrielino NRT

Trail traffic: Moderate—heavy on Brown Mountain Road until El Prieto turnoff, very light to Brown Mountain and down Ken Burton, heavy on Gabrielino National Recreation Trail

Trail surface: Approximately 40% singletrack, 50% fire roads, 10% paved roads; fire roads hard-packed and dry; singletrack loose and mostly dry

Riding time: 3–5 hours

Access: Sunrise—sunset, 7 days

Maps: USGS 7.5-minute quad: Pasadena

Special comments: Be prepared for extreme heat and sun exposure with plenty of sunblock and water.

GPS TRAILHEAD COORDINATES (WGS84)

UTM Zone   11S
Easting   392293
Northing   3785907
Latitude   N 34.12'31"
Longitude   W 118.10'09"

BROWN MOUNTAIN/ KEN BURTON LOOP

In Brief

One of many wild rides in the San Gabriel area, this route involves a long, sustained fire-road climb up Brown Mountain Road followed by a very narrow and treacherous descent into Gabrielino Canyon via the Ken Burton singletrack. This ride is not for the faint of heart: the terrain is very technical, making the consequences of a routine crash possibly severe. The Ken Burton Trail isn't well maintained, so it can be clogged with dense foliage in the spring and early summer. If you are sensitive to poison oak, avoid the area completely and stick to the scenic Brown Mountain Road for an out-and-back. In addition, this area often has poor air quality, so check the news for smog forecasts if this is an issue for you.

Description

The Brown Mountain/Ken Burton Loop is recommended only for mountain bikers of the hardier variety who don't mind getting their feet wet and carrying their bike over technical terrain. Take two to three quarts of water and a nutrition bar or snack. If the weather is hot, start the ride early to avoid experiencing heat exhaustion on the sunny Brown Mountain Fire Road.

From the parking lot, the first 1.5 miles of the ride are paved and will usually be populated with day hikers visiting Gabrielino Canyon. Follow the clear and well-marked signs to Brown Mountain Road. The relentless first 2.5 miles of the climb can be humbling if you're not in good shape. Eventually, the trail flattens a little bit, giving you a breather and a chance to look around and appreciate the

DIRECTIONS

From I-210, take the Arroyo Windsor exit and head north 0.8 miles; park in the large lot on your left. The entrance to the park lies just north of this lot at the end of Windsor Drive.

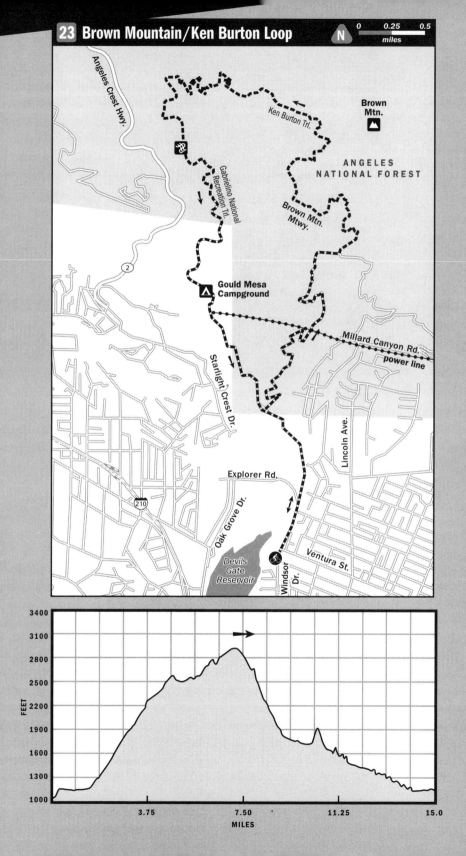

0   0.25   0.5
N
miles

Angeles Crest Hwy.

Ken Burton Trl.

Brown Mtn.

Gabrielino National Recreation Trl.

ANGELES
NATIONAL FOREST

Brown Mtn. Mtwy.

Gould Mesa
Campground

Millard Canyon Rd.
power line

Starlight Crest Dr.

Lincoln Ave.

Explorer Rd.

Oak Grove Dr.

Ventura St.

Devils
Gate
Reservoir

Windsor Dr.

3400
3100
2800
2500
2200
1900
1600
1300
1000

FEET

3.75   7.50   11.25   15.0
MILES

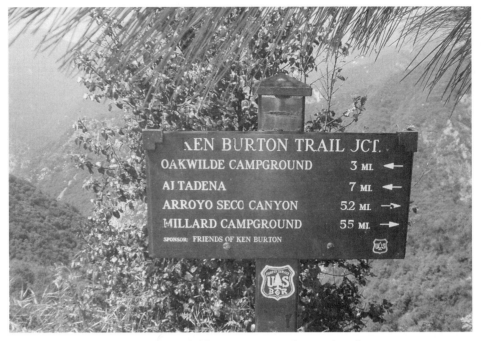

One of the few readable signs in Angeles National Forest

scenery. Roughly 2.7 miles from the start of Brown Mountain Road, you'll see a trail going down to your right and a U.S. Forest Service (USFS) sign on your left. If you were riding the famed El Prieto singletrack, you would turn right here. Instead, continue up Brown Mountain Road toward Arroyo Seco Canyon.

Another 2.6 miles up the Brown Mountain Fire Road, you'll reach the Ken Burton trailhead, which is clearly marked with a USFS sign and is directly at the end of Brown Mountain Road. This is the highest point of the ride, at 2,900 feet, so you may want to sit down, inhale the mountain air, and take in the scenery. You'll see panoramic views of Brown Mountain to the east, Arroyo Seco Canyon to the north, and the city of Los Angeles to the south. Once you're rested and rehydrated, drop your seat post a few inches and charge down the Ken Burton singletrack.

Built specifically for mountain bikers, the Ken Burton Trail immediately earns its fat-tire badge: here you descend a piece of pure SoCal singletrack heaven. The first half mile is largely flat, with minor ascents and descents, after which you'll find yourself staring across a huge void with Arroyo Seco Creek at the bottom. In the next 1.3 miles, you'll lose roughly 1,000 feet of altitude and encounter numerous tight, challenging switchbacks. Agility is key in this section, and no amount of suspension travel will help you overcome obstacles this trail presents. A little too much speed and a wandering front tire will send you tumbling over the hillside, and not enough velocity could yield the same results. The only sounds you'll hear on this section are birds, the clicking of your freewheel, the gurgling creek below, and the whine of sport-bike engines on the Angeles Crest Highway on the other side of the canyon.

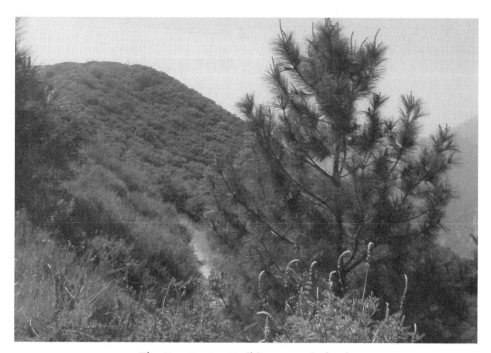

The Ken Burton Trail is narrow indeed.

The Ken Burton Trail ends at Brown Mountain Road, approximately 2 miles after its start, and joins the Gabrielino National Recreation Trail (NRT) in the Arroyo Seco watershed. Turn left here and begin the mellow descent on the Gabrielino NRT, which meanders along both sides of Arroyo Seco Creek. You'll cross the creek several times, so prepare to get wet. Hiking will be an inevitable part of the experience because many parts of the Gabrielino are too rocky and/or sandy to pedal. The trail is sometimes difficult to follow, so you may find yourself at a large man-made waterfall wondering what you did wrong. This is a common error. Don't panic—just backtrack an eighth of a mile, keeping an eye out on your right for the trail, which goes up the east side of the canyon briefly, circumventing the huge waterfall.

After the waterfall, the trail drops to parallel the creek for the rest of the way, getting easier and wider as you go, until it becomes paved. Day hikers and horseback riders frequent this area, so be wary. When you pass the entrance to Brown Mountain Road, give yourself a pat on the back, because you've just completed one of the most challenging rides in LA County.

After the Ride

For beer aficionados and the malnourished, pay a visit to The Stuffed Sandwich at 1145 East Las Tunas Drive in nearby San Gabriel; (626) 285-9161. For a larger appetite, try Zeke's Smokehouse BBQ at 2209 Honolulu Avenue in Montrose; (818) 206-8947. It has a casual atmosphere and serves ridiculously tasty cuisine that will thoroughly alleviate any carbohydrate, protein, or fat deficiencies.

24

BROWN MOUNTAIN/ EL PRIETO

In Brief

El Prieto is probably the most popular singletrack route in LA County. Its considerable technical difficulty and closeness to LA make it attractive to the masses. Although this has become a regular haunt for downhillers, don't be intimidated on the way up Brown Mountain Road by the their big bikes, full-face helmets, and body armor—any skilled rider on any type of mountain bike can clean this descent. You can even do this ride if you're a novice as long as you're prepared to dismount and walk several sections. The heavy traffic this trail receives has damaged it, so all riders should avoid cutting switchbacks and blazing their own lines.

Description

This is the prime after-work ride of the San Gabriel Mountains because the trailhead is centrally located and requires only a two-hour commitment. If you choose to do this route in the summer, don't hesitate to start the ride late, as it can be extremely hot. Even the most experienced riders can find themselves crippled by the heat, along with the smog that can plague the area, on the climb up Brown Mountain Road.

After slathering on copious amounts of your favorite UV blocker and filling your hydration pack to capacity, hit the road. Head north from the parking lot, and continue beyond the end of the arroyo to the gated road marked with a sign for the Gabrielino National Recreation Trail.

KEY AT-A-GLANCE INFORMATION

Length: 8 miles

Configuration: Loop

Technical difficulty: 5

Aerobic difficulty: 3

Scenery: Arroyo Seco, Fern Canyon, Brown Mountain, Millard Canyon, Los Angeles

Exposure: 50% exposed to sunshine

Trail traffic: Moderate–heavy on weekdays, very heavy on weekends

Trail surface: Varies from dry hard-pack to loose and rocky surface—20% singletrack

Riding time: 2–3 hours

Access: Sunrise–sunset, 7 days a week

Maps: USGS 7.5-minute quad: Pasadena

Special comments: Check smog forecasts, and be wary of extreme heat.

GPS TRAILHEAD COORDINATES (WGS84)

UTM Zone 11S
Easting 392365
Northing 3786165
Latitude N 34.12'39"
Longitude W 118.10'06"

DIRECTIONS

From I-210, take the Arroyo Windsor exit and head north 0.8 miles; park in the large lot on your left. The entrance to the park lies just north of this lot at the end of Windsor Drive.

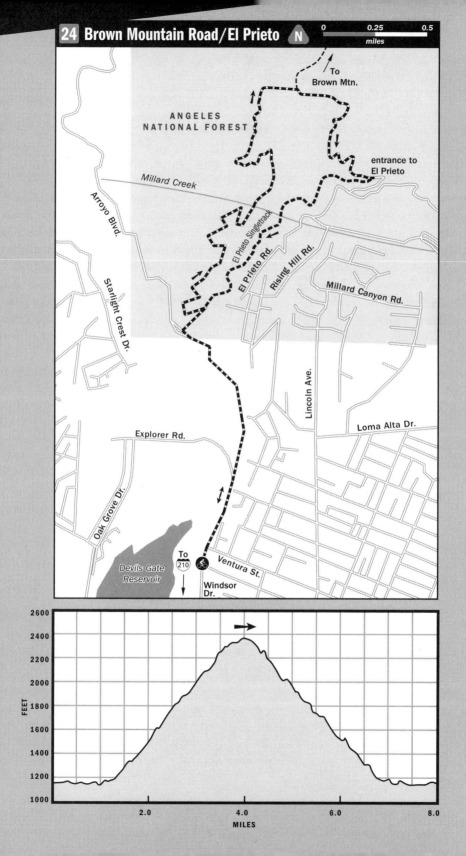

ANGELES
NATIONAL FOREST

To
Brown Mtn.

entrance to
El Prieto

Millard Creek

Arroyo Blvd.

El Prieto Singletrack

El Prieto Rd.

Rising Hill Rd.

Millard Canyon Rd.

Starlight Crest Dr.

Lincoln Ave.

Loma Alta Dr.

Explorer Rd.

Oak Grove Dr.

To
210

Ventura St.

Devils Gate
Reservoir

Windsor
Dr.

FEET

2600
2400
2200
2000
1800
1600
1400
1200
1000

2.0   4.0   6.0   8.0
MILES

Spin away the first 1.4 miles to the turnoff for Brown Mountain Road, a clearly signposted right turn. After roughly 500 feet of dirt, you'll see the lower entrance of El Prieto Trail. Save El Prieto for later and continue up Brown Mountain Road. Start thinking about baseball here so you can ignore the burning sensation in your lungs and legs as you start your quest to slay nearly 1,000 feet of elevation over the next 2.5 miles. If you're unlucky enough to hit this spot on a still, obscenely hot summer day, try to maintain the rpm's to keep your radiators from boiling over, and be prepared to swat away some bugs.

Oddly, many riders choose to bomb down Brown Mountain Road instead of El Prieto, so watch out for reckless riders and avoid hugging the blind corners on your way to the summit. After 2.5 miles of climbing, a small grove of pine trees and an open gate will appear, marking a fork where you will turn right after a snack and a breather, if necessary. Turn right at the fork for a mild 1-mile fire-road descent with a short climb. Keep an eye out for the upper entrance to El Prieto Trail, which will be marked with a small sign, on your right.

You'll immediately see why this trail scores a 5 for technical difficulty. This 1.5-mile descent through a shaded ravine is very steep and full of rocky obstacles and includes countless near-impassable switchbacks. In addition to the technical subtleties are a few places where the trail divides briefly and then rejoins itself, giving the rider several lines to choose from on the way down. At a couple of spots, the trail gets very narrow, with disastrous falls for careless front-tire wandering. Be careful and walk the bike through these sections—you can't be airlifted out of here too easily because of the large oak trees. It's easy to be taken by the scenic wonder of this spot—the gurgling creek snaking through the hillside, amid eroded sandstone boulders seemingly held in place by nothing more that the odd twig or oak root, is mesmerizing, to say the least. It's no wonder the old-school cyclists are very critical of the new school and their perceived destruction and lack of respect for the trail's delicate state. Curb erosion by staying on the trail and not skidding your rear tire around every turn so your kids can enjoy this place, too.

If you finish El Prieto early enough and you've got energy to spare, don't hesitate to take another lap to see if you can decrease your dab coefficient on your second run. If you're thoroughly spent, take a left and head back to your car.

After the Ride

For beer aficionados and the malnourished, pay a visit to The Stuffed Sandwich at 1145 East Las Tunas Drive in nearby San Gabriel; (626) 285-9161. For a larger appetite, try Zeke's Smokehouse BBQ at 2209 Honolulu Avenue in Montrose; (818) 206-8947. It has a casual atmosphere and serves ridiculously tasty cuisine that will thoroughly alleviate any carbohydrate, protein, or fat deficiencies.

KEY AT-A-GLANCE INFORMATION

Length: 9.5 miles

Configuration: Figure-8

Technical difficulty: 4

Aerobic difficulty: 4

Scenery: Echo Mountain, Millard Canyon, Mount Lowe, Muir Peak

Exposure: 80% exposed to sunshine

Trail traffic: Moderate on weekdays, heavy on weekends

Trail surface: Dry, loose, and boulder-strewn on the descent, dry and hard-packed on the way up

Riding time: 2.5–3.5 hours

Access: Sunrise–sunset, 7 days a week

Maps: USGS 7.5-minute quads: Pasadena, Mount Wilson

Special comments: A Forest Adventure Pass is required for each parked vehicle. These can be purchased for $5 from various private vendors and ranger stations listed at **www.fs.fed.us/r5/ sanbernardino/ap/welcome.shtml.**

GPS TRAILHEAD COORDINATES (WGS84)

UTM Zone   11S
Easting   395846
Northing   3786602
Latitude   N 34.12'55"
Longitude   W 118.07.50

MOUNT LOWE RAILWAY/ SAM MERRILL TRAIL/ SUNSET TRAIL

In Brief

This route has it all: a challenging, lung- and leg-burning ascent, great views, numerous plaques with historical factoids to read on the way up, and a heart-stopping descent with endless technical challenges and sheer cliffs nearby to test your intestinal fortitude. The Mount Lowe Railway, with the descents on Sam Merrill and Sunset trails, will challenge riders of all skill levels and must be experienced by everyone.

Safety Message

Novice riders be wary: the entire trail is exposed to many steep drop-offs and cliffs. It may be best to avoid this trail entirely if your technical skills aren't up to par.

Description

The Mount Lowe Railway is what remains of an old railroad track that was built before the turn of the 20th century and that remained in operation until the mid-1930s. It transported travelers to various points of interest at the summit and to two fancy mountain chalets. Few remnants of the actual tracks remain, but the ruins of some of the facilities still stand at the

DIRECTIONS

From I-210 in Altadena, take the Lake Avenue exit, and head north about 3.5 miles to the dead end and Loma Alta Drive. Turn left onto Loma Alta; continue 1 mile, and make a right onto Chaney Trail. Ascend Chaney Trail about 1 mile, watching for the gateway to Mount Lowe Railway on your right before making a hard downhill left turn. Park on the shoulder near the gate, and display your Forest Adventure Pass.

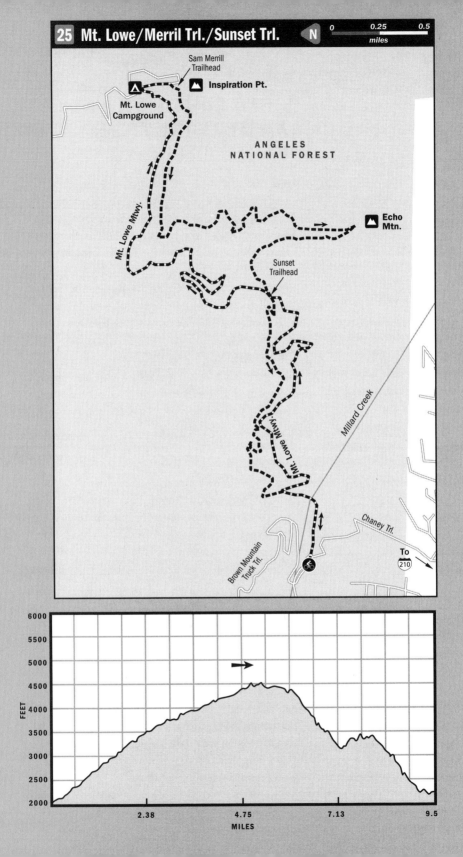

0   0.25   0.5
miles

Sam Merrill
Trailhead

Inspiration Pt.

Mt. Lowe
Campground

A N G E L E S
N A T I O N A L   F O R E S T

Mt. Lowe Mtwy.

Echo
Mtn.

Sunset
Trailhead

Millard Creek

Mt. Lowe Mtwy.

Chaney Trl.

Brown Mountain
Truck Trl.

To
210

FEET

6000
5500
5000
4500
4000
3500
3000
2500
2000

2.38   4.75   7.13   9.5

MILES

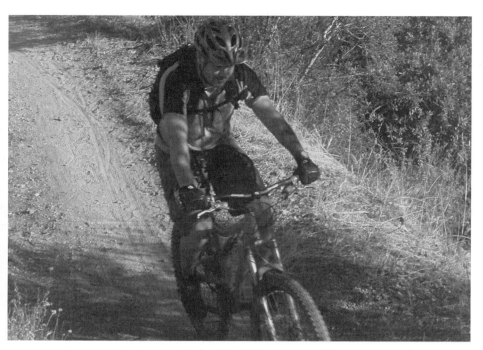

Jason Tuttle breaks in his new Heckler.

summit. Don't worry—the many plaques alongside the railway will answer any questions you have about the history of this site.

After you've geared up with 100 ounces of water and pocketed your cell phone (this is a dangerous ride, remember), start spinning up the railway. Numerous informative plaques will start to appear after the first mile, but don't read all of them because you have to gain nearly 3,500 feet over the next 5 miles. Ouch! As long as it isn't a hot, buggy day, it's an easy ascent (if there is such a thing) because it's mostly paved, albeit very steep in some sections.

Resist the temptation to stop when you get tired. Stopping only makes it more difficult because you lose the invaluable warmth that has built up in your legs. Even after a measly 5-minute rest, your legs will cool significantly and the pain will be much more severe when you start again. Just keep spinning and try to think about something other than your fatigue. Eventually, the pain will go away.

At the 5-mile mark, you've reached the Mount Lowe Campground, which sits atop the ruins of the Mount Lowe Tavern. This is a great place to refuel your body for the demanding descent that lies ahead. After you've hydrated yourself and munched on gimmicky exercise foods, pedal up the road a quarter mile farther to the entrance to Sam Merrill Trail, marked by a weathered sign on the right.

The beginning of the Sam Merrill Trail has too many impassable technical obstructions to allow you to build any kind of momentum, which gets kind of frustrating. You'll soon find that Sam Merrill Trail isn't an easy bomb—you're always on the edge, constantly negotiating sharp turns, boulders, and ruts. It's very demanding. In fact, a five-minute rest is recommended here more than on the way up Mount Lowe Railway. You are too far from help to risk an injury resulting from fatigue getting the best of you.

Take a hard right on Echo Mountain Trail at the 7.3-mile mark, which is the top of Echo Mountain, the site of the ruins of the old White City Resort. Echo Mountain Trail traverses Las Flores Canyon for 0.8 miles, with many steep cliffs on the left along the way. A word of advice: look where you want to go instead of where you don't and you won't have any problems.

At the 8-mile mark, go left on the Mount Lowe Railway for a few feet, and then turn right to descend Sunset Trail, which is slightly less hairy than Sam Merrill but very technical nonetheless. After oodles of grin-inspiring singletrack action, take a left roughly 9.6 miles from the start to go back to the Mount Lowe Railway and avoid descending all the way to the Millard Picnic Area.

Congratulations: you've just completed the toughest 10 miles of riding, bar none, in all of SoCal. You now have bragging rights, great stories to tell, and a higher IQ score—courtesy of all the informative plaques you read on the way up.

After the Ride

Since you just revisited history on the old Mount Lowe Railway, you might want to return to the days when soul food was considered healthy—stop at the award-winning Big Mamma's Rib Shack at 1453 North Lake Avenue in Pasadena; (626) 797-1792. If that sort of free living alarms you, try Orean Health Express at 817 North Lake Avenue; (626) 794-0861.

26

ECHO MOUNTAIN/LOWER SAM MERRILL TRAIL

KEY AT-A-GLANCE INFORMATION

Length: 7.2 miles

Configuration: Loop

Technical difficulty: 4

Aerobic difficulty: 3

Scenery: Echo Mountain, Los Angeles, Millard Canyon

Exposure: 90% exposed to sunshine

Trail traffic: Moderate–heavy on weekdays, heavy on weekends

Trail surface: Varies from pavement to loose and rocky surface to hardpack with embedded rocks—40% singletrack

Riding time: 1.5–2.5 hours

Access: Sunrise–sunset, 7 days a week

Maps: USGS 7.5-minute quad: Pasadena, Mount Wilson

Special comments: The singletrack descent on Lower Sam Merrill Trail has numerous disastrous drops alongside it. Novice riders should avoid this trail.

GPS TRAILHEAD COORDINATES (WGS84)

UTM Zone   11S
Easting   394275
Northing   3786567
Latitude   N 34.12'53"
Longitude   W 118.08'52"

In Brief

To be such a short route, the Echo Mountain/Sam Merrill loop really packs a technical and aerobic punch. With the perfect blend of scenery, vigorous climbing, vertigo-inspiring cliffs, and challenging switchbacks, this may be the perfect after-work ride because it can be finished in less than two hours. If it does become part of your post-clock-out regimen, don't ever lose respect for the danger that this trail presents—complacency can cause severe injuries and even death on the Lower Sam Merrill Trail.

Description

To complete the bulk of climbing at the beginning rather than the end, start somewhere near the intersection of Chaney Trail and Loma Alta Drive. Get ready for a lot of work—you'll gain nearly 2,000 feet of elevation over the next 3.5 miles. This is a granny-gear climb in many places, so all but the strongest single speeders may find themselves walking a lot.

After about a mile, turn right at the first intersection, go around the gate, and start ascending what remains of the old Mount Lowe Railway. There's not much left of this railroad track, which many years ago carried men and women of leisure up the hill for weekend vacations, so don't waste your time looking for ruins on this route. You can see them only in the upper section, which is not included on this route. Take solace in the fact that modern men and women of leisure, like yourself, burn calories instead of coal to make the ascent.

DIRECTIONS

From I-210 in Altadena, take the Lake Avenue exit, and head north about 3.5 miles to the dead end and Loma Alta Drive. Turn left onto Loma Alta; continue 1 mile, and turn right onto Chaney Trail. Park at the first available spot alongside the road.

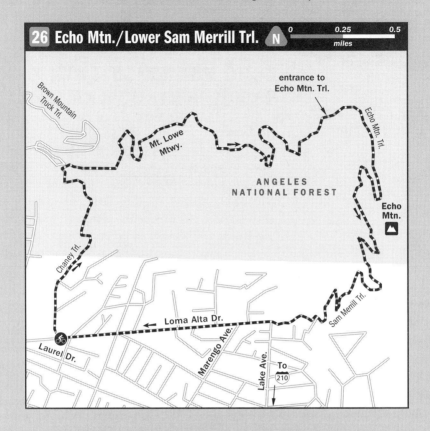

26 **Echo Mtn./Lower Sam Merrill Trl.** N

0   0.25   0.5
miles

entrance to
Echo Mtn. Trl.

Brown Mountain
Truck Trl.

Mt. Lowe
Mtwy.

Echo Mtn. Trl.

ANGELES
NATIONAL FOREST

Echo
Mtn.

Chaney Trl.

Sam Merrill Trl.

Loma Alta Dr.

Marengo Ave.

Lake Ave.

Laurel Dr.

To
210

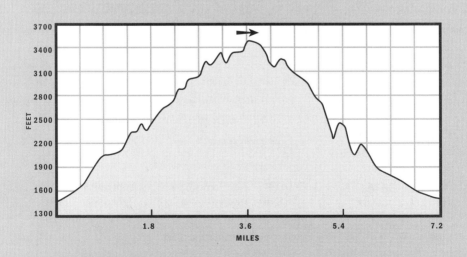

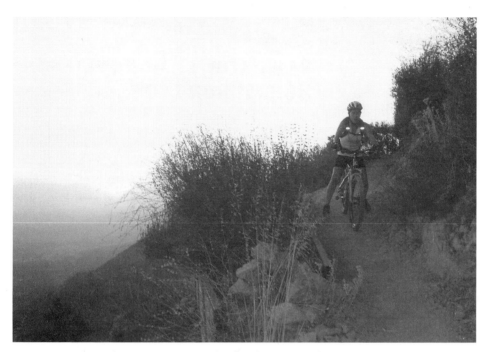

Echo Mountain isn't for newbies—Stephanie agrees.

As you make your way up, your sweat-stung eyes will take in such scenic elements as Millard Canyon to your left and Mount Lowe above. Your knobbies will be out of their element until you leave pavement for the descent on Echo Mountain Trail, which appears as a right turn about 3.5 miles from the Chaney Trail–Loma Alta Drive intersection.

As you traverse Las Flores Canyon to Echo Mountain, it will be immediately apparent why this route description includes so many ominous warnings. On your right side, nearly the whole way, are a plethora of potential catastrophes, from the occasional bone-snapping 15-foot cliff to several seemingly endless near-vertical chutes into the canyon below. The trail itself, however, is flat, packed, and lacking the rocky obstacles so prevalent on the other trails in this area. This characteristic, as well as its closeness to civilization, makes this trail attractive to joggers, dog walkers, and hikers. You'll see many of them all the way down, so stay wary and courteous.

After about 0.7 miles of mild descending, you can, if curious, take a spur out to the ruins of the old White City Resort perched atop Echo Mountain. Otherwise, turn right to descend Lower Sam Merrill Trail, which is signposted. This trail continues the trend established by Echo Mountain Trail—it's a wide, flat, flowing singletrack with few technical obstacles and many disastrous drop-offs. If you've timed your ride perfectly and the sun is starting to set, you'll see the sun ablaze over the Verdugo Mountains.

After about 6.25 miles, you'll be dumped out onto the street; turn right and begin the easy mile-long steady descent on Loma Alta Drive. Once you get back to your car, consult a local realtor to find lodging in the Pasadena-Altadena area, surely the best place to live for the SoCal fat-tire enthusiast.

27

SAN GABRIEL MOUNTAINS: MOUNT ZION LOOP

KEY AT-A-GLANCE INFORMATION

Length: 13.7 miles

Configuration: Loop

Technical difficulty: 5

Aerobic difficulty: 4

Scenery: Santa Anita Canyon, Winter Creek, Mount Zion, Mount Wilson, Clamshell Peak, Santa Anita Dam

Exposure: 80% shaded

Trail traffic: Light on weekdays, moderate on weekends

Trail surface: Varies from loose and dry surface, to hard-packed clay with embedded boulders—55% singletrack

Riding time: 4–6 hours

Access: Sunrise–sunset, 7 days a week

Maps: USGS 7.5-minute quad: Mount Wilson

GPS TRAILHEAD COORDINATES (WGS84)

UTM Zone   11S
Easting   405533
Northing   3784283
Latitude   N 34.11'43"
Longitude   W 118.01'31"

In Brief

You may be wondering why a measly 14-mile ride with 4,200 feet of elevation gain would require a four- to six-hour commitment. The Mount Zion Loop is for true adventurers: the soft need not apply. Hiking and biking go hand in hand on this journey because much of the trail is too overgrown, narrow, and precarious to pedal. Those afflicted with bouts of vertigo will find themselves frozen in awe at the many exposed sections of loose, tire-width singletrack on the described route. Courage and skill earn great dividends; Upper Winter Creek Trail, where ridable, is the sort of priceless terrain that mountain bikers dream about, and it affords you the rare opportunity to leave the sunblock at home—the trail is almost completely shaded by lanky oak, sycamore, and pine trees.

Safety Message

This ride is *very* dangerous, so do *not* attempt it alone. Do *not* attempt this ride if you are not an experienced, highly skilled rider, or if you're with anyone who isn't an experienced, highly skilled rider. Do *not* attempt this route with less than seven hours of sunshine remaining in the day. Do *not* attempt this ride without a full assortment of epic ride gear, including but not limited to tons of water, food, tools, a first-aid kit, at least two spare tubes, a patch kit, maps, a cell phone, and a GPS unit. Lastly, do *not* attempt this ride without telling someone exactly where you are going.

DIRECTIONS

From I-210 in Arcadia, take the Santa Anita Avenue exit, and head north about 1.6 miles. Park in the residential neighborhood below the gate just inside the entrance to Santa Anita Canyon Road.

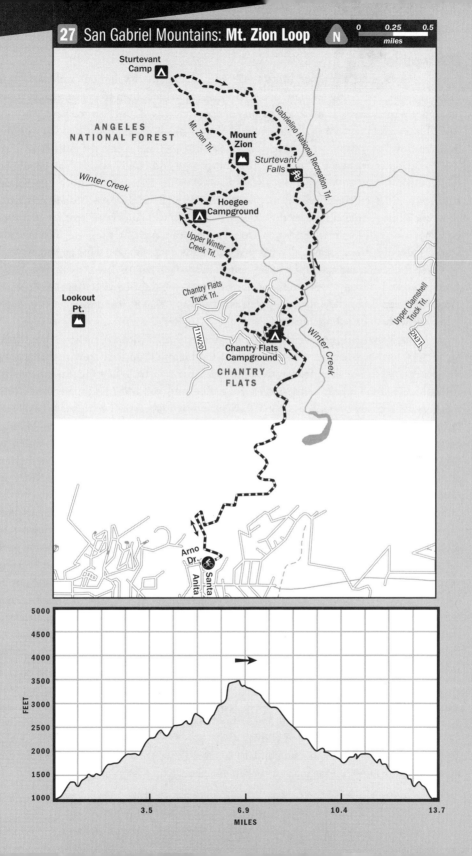

N

0   0.25   0.5
miles

Sturtevant
Camp

Gabrielino National Recreation Trl.

ANGELES
NATIONAL FOREST

Mt. Zion Trl.

**Mount
Zion**

Sturtevant
Falls

Winter Creek

Hoegee
Campground

Upper Winter
Creek Trl.

Chantry Flats
Truck Trl.

Lookout
Pt.

11W20

Upper Clamshell
Truck Trl.

2N31

**Chantry Flats
Campground**

Winter Creek

CHANTRY
FLATS

Arno
Dr.

Santa
Anita

FEET

5000
4500
4000
3500
3000
2500
2000
1500
1000

3.5   6.9   10.4   13.7
MILES

Description

If having to ascend the 3 paved miles to Chantry Flats bothers you, don't undertake this route. If you're not strong enough for a 1,200-foot road climb, then you're surely not ready for Upper Winter Creek Trail, so the pavement does the work of thinning the herd. But consider this: why let the roadies have all the fun? Santa Anita Canyon Road is popular with the thin-tire crowd of Arcadia for good reason—it's a blast, and very scenic the entire way.

Once you arrive at the Chantry Flats Campground and ranger station, you should be thoroughly warmed up for what lies ahead. Just follow the signs to the clearly signposted Upper Winter Creek Trail, which is reached by turning right off the paved road that ascends above the campground at roughly the 3.5-mile mark. You will quickly see that my ominous warnings are anything but hype as you ascend a razor-thin path, skirting the hillside while ignoring the disastrous slides and cliffs that lead to the dark, spooky ravine etched by Winter Creek far below. You can take a little comfort in the fact that, in case of a fall, you would simply descend Winter Creek to its convergence with the Gabrielino National Recreation Trail (NRT) rather than trying to claw your way back up—that is, if you were lucky enough to survive without crippling injuries.

Although the trail gets hairier as you progress, the grade doesn't get any more severe before you start the brief descent to the Hoegee Campground, adjacent to Winter Creek. At this point, cross the creek and follow the signs to Mount Zion Trail. Now the real fun begins. Although the climb is only a little more than a mile long, you won't find many opportunities to pedal because of steepness, thick foliage, and lack of traction, so this is hike-a-bike. However, this section of trail does get occasional maintenance and repair, so it could be in better shape by the time you read this. Resist the urge to turn back, and trudge your way past the Mount Zion Trail spur to Sturtevant Camp, which consists of a boarded red cabin at roughly the 7.25-mile mark. At this point, you will merge with the Gabrielino NRT and head down the canyon.

For the rest of the way, the Gabrielino snakes through various old settlements that served as base camps for hikers and outdoorsmen around the end of the 19th and beginning of the 20th centuries. Don't be alarmed if you see people living in some of them—the park still leases a few of these cabins to a handful of people who have improved them over the years to livable condition. The Gabrielino descent provides a welcome break from the formidable combo of Upper Winter Creek and Mount Zion—most of the Gabrielino lacks major trail obstructions and technical obstacles. At roughly the 9-mile mark, the Gabrielino leaves creek level and skirts the hillside for a while, exposing a few nasty drops and cliffs along the way that are reminiscent of those you encountered earlier; however, a more manageable riding surface here makes avoiding death slightly easier.

As you close in on the 10-mile mark, the Gabrielino parallels the creek again to take you past more old settlements, the last of which, Robert's Camp, appears at roughly the 10.4-mile mark. A plaque at this site gives a brief historical blurb about the settlement. Just beyond the plaque, turn right and climb a short, paved grinder back up to Chantry Flats. Then stop, take a deep breath, and bomb back down Santa Anita Canyon Road to your car, knowing you're lucky to have made it back in one piece.

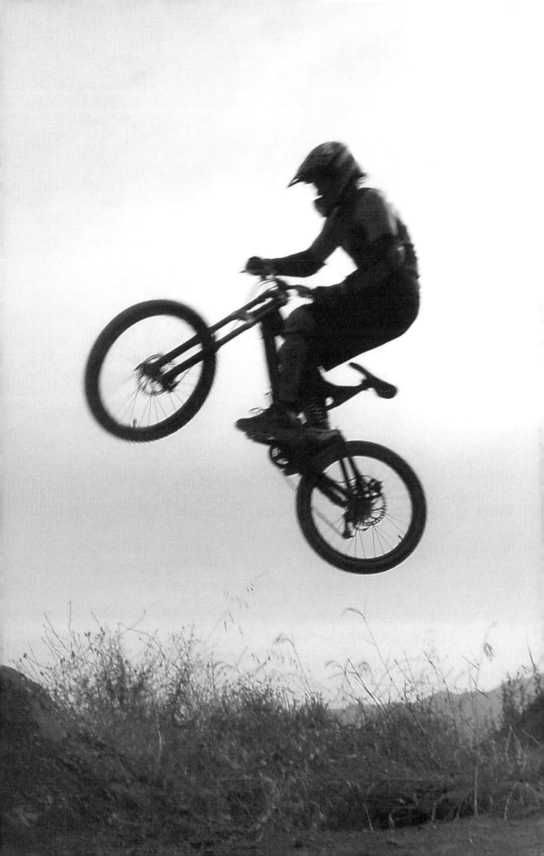

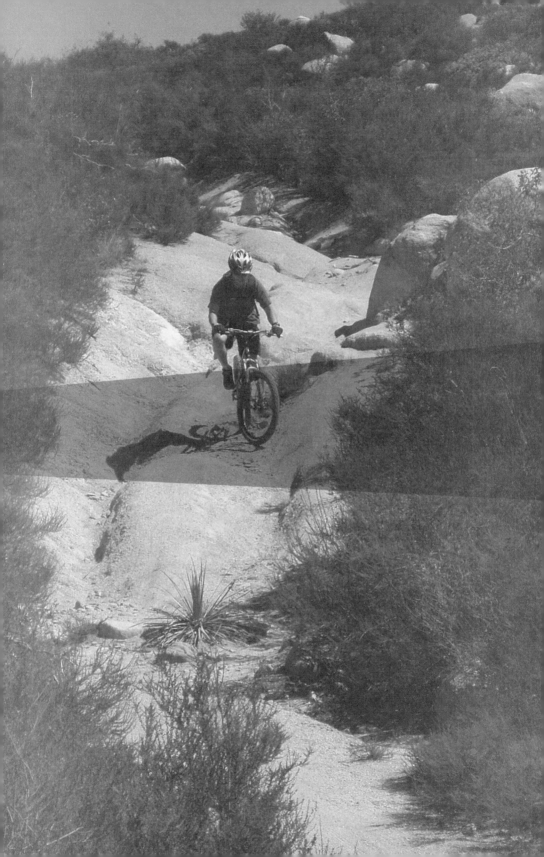

LOS ANGELES COUNTY

28

COLDWATER CANYON PARK

Length: 3.1 miles

Configuration: Loop

Technical difficulty: 1

Aerobic difficulty: 2

Scenery: Iredell Canyon

Exposure: 40% exposed to sunshine

Trail traffic: Moderate–heavy during weekdays, heavy on weekends

Trail surface: Hard-packed fire roads—no singletrack

Riding time: Less than 1 hour

Access: Sunrise–sunset, 7 days a week

Maps: USGS 7.5-minute quad: Beverly Hills

Special comments: Masses of pedestrians walk this route.

In Brief

At only 3.1 miles in length, with no technical subtleties, this route barely qualifies as a mountain bike ride. All new mountain bikers, however, need short routes like this to get "broken in." Added features include the Tree People park facilities and this park's central location, right between West Hollywood and Studio City. Is 3.1 miles not enough for you? Try doing six laps!

Description

Once you've found the somewhat elusive Tree People parking lot and park facilities, carry your bike down a stairway at the north side of the lot, and turn left onto the first trail that comes into view. This shredded-wood trail is used mainly by pedestrians, so keep your velocity low. Shortly, the trail winds around 180 degrees, assuming the name Oak Trail. Heading west on Oak Trail, you'll pass the Mark Taper outdoor amphitheater on your left. After a few more pedal strokes, make a left turn onto Betty Dearing Trail.

The 1.3-mile Betty Dearing Trail is composed of hard-packed dry dirt and entirely free of technical subtleties, which is a relief for novice riders and dull for those more skilled. After a little while, the trail is paved, though it's still called a trail. Roughly 1.75

GPS TRAILHEAD
COORDINATES (WGS84)
UTM Zone 11S
Easting 370330
Northing 3777373
Latitude N 34.07'45"
Longitude W 118.24'22"

DIRECTIONS

From Los Angeles, take Interstate 405 north to the Skirball Center/Mulholland exit. Turn left onto Skirball Center Drive, proceed to Mulholland Drive, and turn right. About 2.2 miles beyond the stoplight at Benedict Canyon Drive, turn left into the "Tree People" parking lot, directly opposite Franklin Canyon Drive. Park your vehicle in this lot.

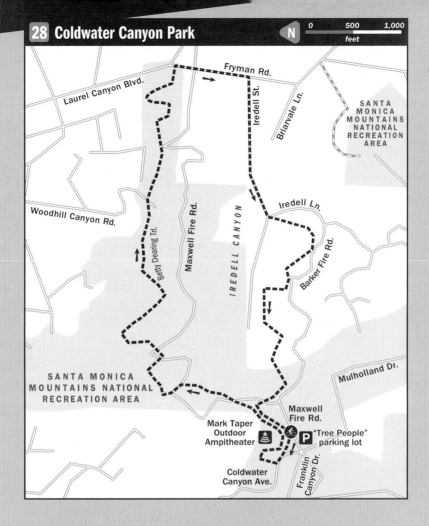

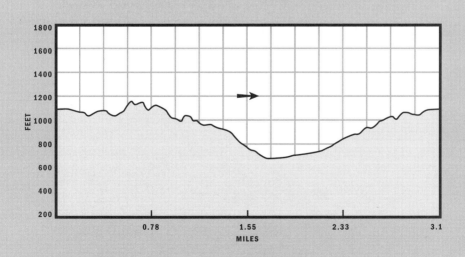

miles along, turn right onto Fryman Road. Make another right onto Iredell Street, followed by another quick right onto Iredell Lane.

At the end of Iredell Lane lies the entrance to another fire road that climbs back to your point of origin, intersecting Betty Dearing Trail once again. Unless you're an absolute newbie, you should be barely breaking a sweat at this point, so I suggest taking at least one or two more laps to facilitate proper calorie burning. It's true that Coldwater Canyon Park doesn't offer much for the seasoned mountain biker—this route is included to turn new people on to the sport and also provide a safe place to hone basic off-road cycling skills. (Remember how many times you fell on your rump when you made the switch to clipless pedals?) You wouldn't be alive to read this today if you made those mistakes on the disastrous Strawberry Peak Trail in the San Gabriel Mountains.

After the Ride

This is LA, remember; you've gotta get with it and learn to like sushi! Get used to eating raw fish at Katsu-Ya at 11980 Ventura Boulevard in Studio City; (818) 985-6976. For a little more ruckus, head to West Hollywood's own Barney's Beanery, at 8447 Santa Monica Boulevard, for beer, sports, and bar food; (323) 654-512

GETTY VIEW TRAIL

In Brief

If you've spent any time in LA, chances are you've been stuck in traffic on the 405 going over the Sepulveda Pass. Adjacent to this mass exodus of road rage–infused commuters lie a few miles of underappreciated, underrated, and often overlooked singletrack. The lack of traffic here may owe to the facts that Getty View Trail was only recently constructed and Casiano Fire Road isn't connected by dirt to the Santa Monica Mountains National Recreation Area. This sliver of mountain bike terrain is totally surrounded by urban development. Nevertheless, it offers the most centrally located fat-tire action in all of LA.

Length: 5.4 miles

Configuration: Loop with short spurs

Technical difficulty: 3

Aerobic difficulty: 2

Scenery: Hoag Canyon, West Los Angeles, Getty Museum, Pacific Ocean

Exposure: 95% exposed to sunshine

Trail traffic: Light on weekdays, moderate on weekends

Trail surface: Dry hardpack with some loose areas—40% singletrack

Riding time: 1 hour

Access: Sunrise–sunset, 7 days a week

Maps: USGS 7.5-minute quad: Beverly Hills

Special comments: Poison oak is present on the lower part of Getty View Trail.

Description

It's maddening to know that a nice piece of singletrack like the Getty View Trail gets so little fat-tire traffic, despite its being so close to the homes of thousands of mountain bikers. Its somewhat mangy, overgrown state is due to the apathy of LA's mountain bike community. Do your part, and ride this trail today!

That's right: mount up, pay the measly $3 parking, and get going. After the first few switchbacks, it becomes apparent that this trail wasn't exactly designed for mountain bikers. Your riding this trail on your rig is tantamount to Paul Bunyan's riding Backbone Trail atop a 40-foot-tall custom bicycle. The turns are very tight, the trail is impossibly narrow—but that's what we live for, right? If we wanted an easy ride, we'd be down on Venice Beach soaking up UV rays on a low rider.

GPS TRAILHEAD COORDINATES (WGS84)

UTM Zone 11S
Easting 363823
Northing 3773855
Latitude N 34.05'48"
Longitude W 118.28'34"

DIRECTIONS

From Los Angeles, take I-405 north toward Sacramento (from the San Fernando Valley, head south); exit at Getty Center Drive. Head north on Sepulveda Boulevard; the Getty View Trail parking lot will soon appear on the right.

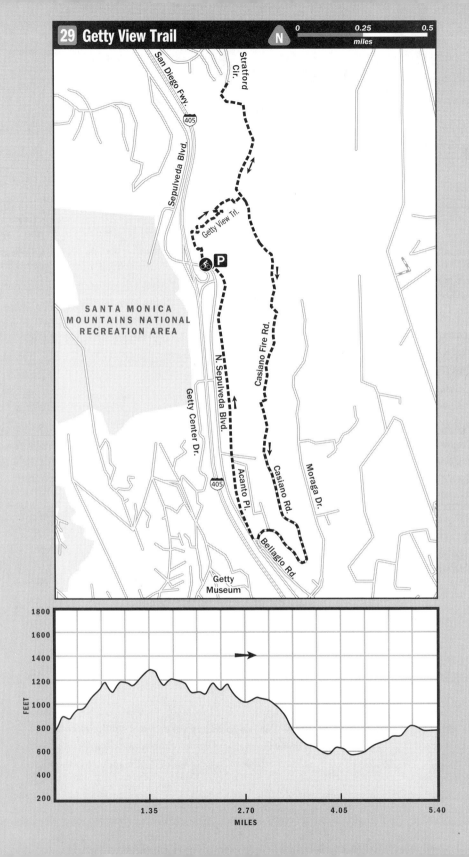

N

0   0.25   0.5
miles

Stratford Cir.

San Diego Fwy.

405

Sepulveda Blvd.

Getty View Trl.

P

SANTA MONICA
MOUNTAINS NATIONAL
RECREATION AREA

N. Sepulveda Blvd.

Casiano Fire Rd.

Getty Center Dr.

405

Acanto Pl.

Casiano Rd.

Moraga Dr.

Bellagio Rd.

Getty
Museum

1800
1600
1400
1200
1000
800
600
400
200

FEET

1.35   2.70   4.05   5.40

MILES

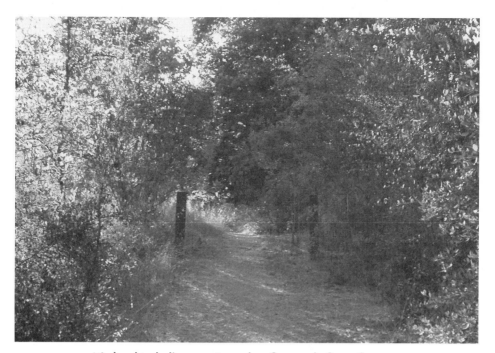

It's hard to believe you're only a few yards from the 405.

You may find yourself carrying your bike a little and getting somewhat frustrated, but the trek ends at 0.8 miles from the start, where it intersects with Casiano Fire Road. Since you have limited terrain to play with on this ride, go left here and spin your way up to the end of the road, where it terminates into a community of fancy homes. Turn around and head back to where you came from, but keep an eye out for a singletrack offshoot that runs along the right side of the road—ride this trail. It's tight but still roomier than Getty View Trail and much more interesting than the fire road. After a quarter of a mile, it reconnects with the fire road, after which you'll pass your point of origin.

You have a choice now: take the easy route and enjoy the views of West LA, the Pacific Ocean, and the Getty Museum on the fire road, or do some more bushwhacking on the singletrack that parallels it. Since your rig was built stout and designed for harsh conditions, go up the singletrack diversion on the left about 2 miles from the start of the ride. It parallels the fire road for a few hundred feet and then reconnects with it briefly, after which you'll see another singletrack veering off from Casiano Road. This one is very steep, requiring a burst of horsepower to the cranks. This last singletrack is 0.7 miles long and will dump you out where Casiano Fire Road ends and becomes the paved, residential Casiano Road.

Roll down Casiano to Sepulveda Boulevard, and turn right. Watch out for angry commuters as you spin the last mile to your vehicle. If they honk or holler harsh epithets, they do so only because they are jealous of your ability to escape the daily rat race. When you get back to your vehicle, tell all your friends about the fun singletrack you discovered in the middle of Babylon, and then pencil your next visit to this place in your date book—Getty View Trail needs to be ridden more.

30

LA TUNA CANYON LOOP

KEY AT-A-GLANCE INFORMATION

Length: 8.7 miles

Configuration: Loop

Technical difficulty: 4

Aerobic difficulty: 3

Scenery: Los Angeles, Verdugo Mountains, San Gabriel Mountains

Exposure: 75% exposed to sunshine

Trail traffic: Moderate–heavy on weekdays, heavy on weekends

Trail surface: Dry with loose and embedded rocks

Riding time: 1.5–2.5 hours

Access: Sunrise–sunset, 7 days a week

Maps: USGS 7.5-minute quad: Burbank

Special comments: Heat and smog can plague this area; check forecasts before proceeding.

GPS TRAILHEAD COORDINATES (WGS84)
UTM Zone 11S
Easting 381206
Northing 3788821
Latitude N 34.14'02"
Longitude W 118.17'26"

In Brief

Without a doubt, the La Tuna Canyon loop provides the most enjoyable ride in the immediate vicinity of Los Angeles. It would be worthy of numerous visits even if it weren't the most centrally located ride in LA, which it is. It has all the key elements of a great loop—an aerobic ascent, fantastic views, and an action-packed singletrack downhill at the end, all of which are packed tightly into a manageable package short enough for an afternoon or before-work visit.

Description

After gearing up, remain wary of speeding vehicles as you ascend La Tuna Canyon Road heading east toward the trailhead. Don't worry—after roughly 1.75 miles you won't smell engine exhaust for the rest of the loop. Turn right into the parking lot, which appears just before the road intersects Interstate 210. Cross the gate at the south end of the parking lot and begin the ascent, which is paved in the beginning and gives way to dirt after a short distance.

After a mellow, winding ascent, you gain roughly 1,600 feet by the 4.4-mile mark, where an absolutely stunning view appears. On a clear day, it's possible to see directly across the skyscrapers of downtown LA all the way to the Pacific Ocean and Catalina Island. Even on a typical smoggy day, the views are

DIRECTIONS

From Los Angeles, take I-5 to Sun Valley, and exit at Sunland Boulevard. Head north on Sunland approximately 0.8 miles, and turn right onto La Tuna Canyon Road. Head east about 3.3 miles, and park on the wide shoulder in front of the small picnic area.

126

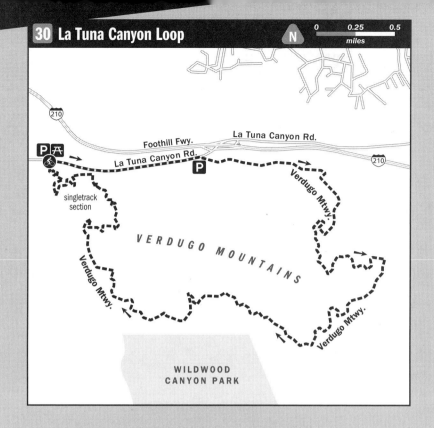

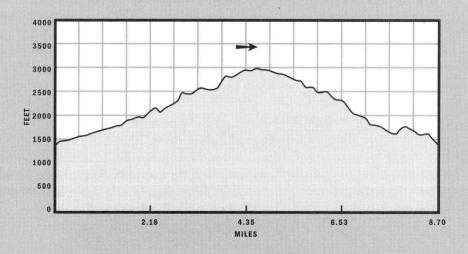

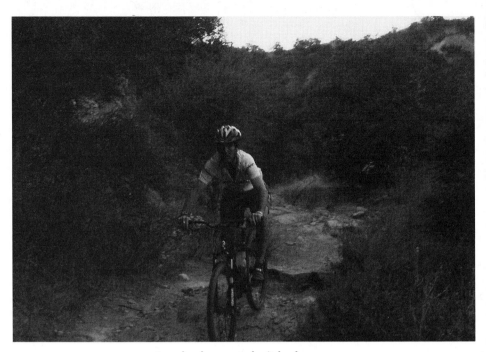

Locals always make it look easy.

breathtaking. After snapping a few pictures, turn right (west), and start the blisteringly fast fire-road descent.

Two miles from the summit and about 6.6 miles from the start of the ride, you'll see a firebreak on the right. The singletrack that takes you back to your car branches off from this firebreak, but it's very easy to miss. Once you've located it, start the tricky, narrow, rocky, rutted descent with a lowered saddle to ensure control and proper weight distribution. The trail from this point includes all the elements of a great singletrack—switchbacks, ruts, and rocks to negotiate—but at a steeper grade many will find uncomfortable yet exciting.

After a few short climbs, you'll drop briefly into a shaded streambed. After a few pedal strokes, the speeding cars of La Tuna Canyon Road (and, hopefully, your car) will come into view. Never again do you have to drive out of your way for great mountain biking in the city of Los Angeles. The La Tuna Canyon loop, seldom included in a SoCal biker's list of top-ten rides, is the best-kept secret in the area.

After the Ride

For rich, carb-replenishing Italian food, visit Giannino, at 2630 Hyperion Avenue in Los Angeles; (323) 664-7979. If you prefer a casual, highly regarded, hole-in-the-wall barbecue outfit, go to Pecos Bill's Bar-B-Q, at 1551 Victory Boulevard in Glendale; (818) 241-2750.

31

PALOS VERDES BLUFFS

KEY AT-A-GLANCE INFORMATION

Length: 5 miles

Configuration: Out-and-back with short spurs

Technical difficulty: 3

Aerobic difficulty: 2

Scenery: Santa Catalina Island, Pacific Ocean, Los Angeles Harbor, Palos Verdes Peninsula

Exposure: 100% exposed to sunshine

Trail traffic: Moderate–heavy

Trail surface: Hard-packed and dry—60% singletrack

Riding time: 1–2 hours

Access: Sunrise–sunset, 7 days a week

Maps: USGS 7.5-minute quad: San Pedro

Special comments: Watch out for the cliffside drop-off at the start of this ride—it's a long way down!

GPS TRAILHEAD COORDINATES (WGS84)

UTM Zone 11S
Easting 376842
Northing 3732041
Latitude N 33.43'16"
Longitude W 118.19'45"

In Brief

The Palos Verdes Bluffs are truly unique—vastly different from any other riding area in Southern California. This small trail network sits atop a high plateau at the end of the Palos Verdes Peninsula, which juts out into the Pacific Ocean toward Santa Catalina Island. The views of the ocean are spectacular, and the mountain biking is nominally challenging, making this a great place for novice riders to get started.

Description

Once you've packed your sunscreen, swimsuit, and maybe a small beach towel (one trail spur literally ends on the beach), roll to the trailhead at the end of Warmouth Street, and follow your nose to the ocean.

The first 0.3 miles of the trail will take your breath away as you marvel at the beauty of the Pacific and Catalina Island and gasp for fear of falling off the edge of the cliff that borders the trail, inches from where your tires contact terra firma. Keep your eye on the trail to avoid death, and spin your way to a couple of picnic tables at 0.5 miles. This is a good place to have a snack and take some pictures—don't worry about snacking early because this is a very casual ride.

Backtrack just more than a tenth of a mile to reach a left turn that will take you up a short hill and

DIRECTIONS

From Los Angeles, head south on I-110, and exit onto Gaffey Street. Go south on Gaffey Street about 2.25 miles, and then turn right onto West 25th Street. Continue about 1.7 miles; then make a left on Anchovy Avenue, followed by a quick right onto Paseo Del Mar, a left onto Stargazer Street, and a right onto Warmouth Street. The trailhead is at the end of Warmouth and is easily visible on the ocean side of the road. Park anywhere on the street.

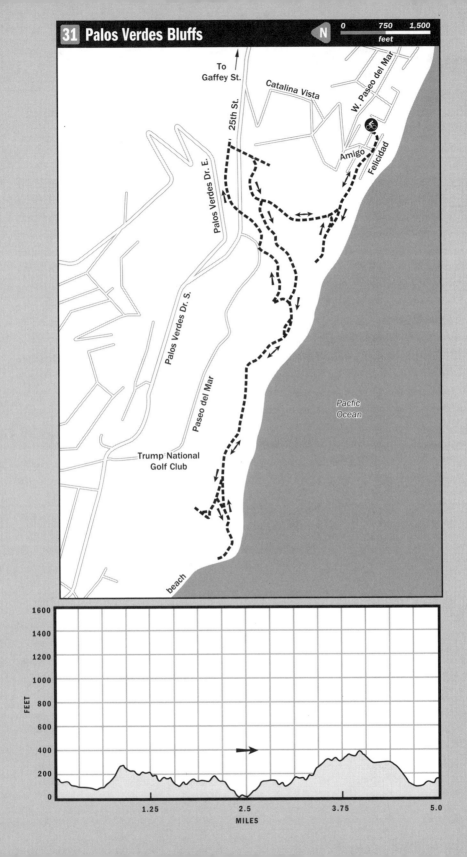

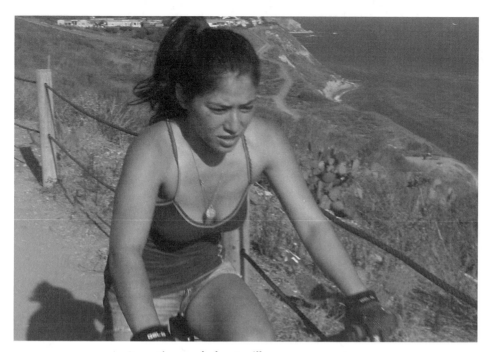

Sometimes a helmet will mess up your tan.

connect with the rest of the Palos Verdes Bluffs trail network. Watch for a singletrack that heads left, back toward the ocean along the hill. Turn left here, and pedal up the singletrack. Eventually, the trail will start to look more groomed, fenced on both sides, but still narrow enough to qualify as singletrack. The views never sour, with the majestic Pacific on your left and an elegant golf course on your right.

Continue on the cliffside trail until you see another trail heading down to the beach, roughly 2 miles from the start. This spur goes directly to the beach; ride your bike all the way down. In SoCal you don't get many opportunities to literally ride on the beach, but here you can—for a short stretch—because the sand is just rocky enough to sustain traction. The trail terminates at a lovely little cove. Park the rigs, do some body surfing, and catch some rays.

Once refreshed, shake the sand off, get back on your bike, and engage the toughest climb of the day back up to the cliffside trail. Now you have a couple of options: you can either backtrack the way you came or goof around by taking the left turn that will appear at roughly the 3.5-mile mark, if you're keeping track. This trail will take you up a hill and over some steps and eventually dump you out onto West 25th Street. Spin on pavement while watching for the first trail entrance that will take you back to the picnic area you encountered early in the ride. Head back to your car, and congratulate your novice riding buddies for completing one of their first bike rides, reassuring them that there are plenty more-challenging routes to enjoy in SoCal.

32

KEY AT-A-GLANCE INFORMATION

Length: 28.5 miles

Configuration: Loop

Technical difficulty: 2

Aerobic difficulty: 5

Scenery: Toyon Bay, Long Point, Mount Orizaba, Mount Banning, Pacific Ocean, Little Harbor, Casino Point, Avalon

Exposure: 100% exposed to sun

Trail traffic: Light every day

Trail surface: Dry hardpack—no singletrack

Riding time: 4–6 hours

Access: Sunrise–sunset, 7 days

Maps: USGS 7.5-minute quads: Santa Catalina North, Santa Catalina South

Special comments: A permit is required to pedal a bicycle anywhere outside Avalon's city limits. You can buy a permit from the Catalina Island Conservancy at the Conservancy House, 125 Claressa Avenue in Avalon, for $20, plus a $40 deposit that's refunded after the pass is returned; (310) 510-2595. Passes will not be issued if your bike doesn't have knobby tires or you don't have a helmet.

GPS TRAILHEAD COORDINATES (WGS84)

W UTM Zone 11S

Easting 375833

Northing 3683422

Latitude N 33.20'50"

Longitude W 118.20'04"

CATALINA ISLAND: AVALON TO LITTLE HARBOR LOOP

In Brief

On paper, mountain biking Santa Catalina Island appears bittersweet. It may seem that the "hassles" involved—the boat ride, $20 passes, and bike inspection—could overshadow the joys of riding the island. Nothing could be further from the truth. Aside from the riding appeal—challenging climbs, breathtaking ocean views, clean air, and unparalleled tranquility—a certain inexplicable "magic" about Catalina becomes apparent only after you get there. Riders of the downhill and freeride set will not have their adrenaline thirsts quenched because there is no technical riding or legal singletrack anywhere on this route or the island as a whole. All the terrain is dirt road. The Avalon to Little Harbor Loop is, however, a climber's delight and, with nearly 5,800 feet of elevation gain, not to be taken lightly by riders in less than adequate cardiovascular condition. Those less inclined toward monstrous aerobic output should opt for the shorter and less demanding East End Loop (see page 134).

Safety Message

You have a very good chance of encountering bison on this route. For the most part, they are harmless—just approach them slowly and respectfully, and they will get out of your way.

DIRECTIONS

After arriving at Catalina Island by boat, helicopter, or plane, make your way to the north end of the oceanfront walk in Avalon, ride left up Marilla Avenue, and then turn right onto Vieudlou Avenue, followed by a left onto Stage Road. At the top of Stage Road, you will see a gate (Hogsback Gate) on your left; the route starts just beyond the gate.

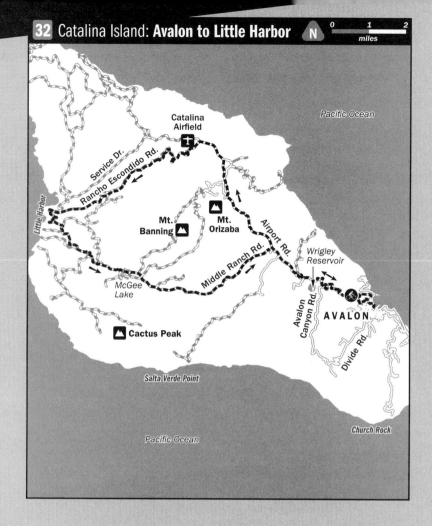

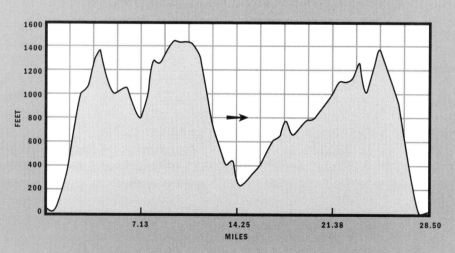

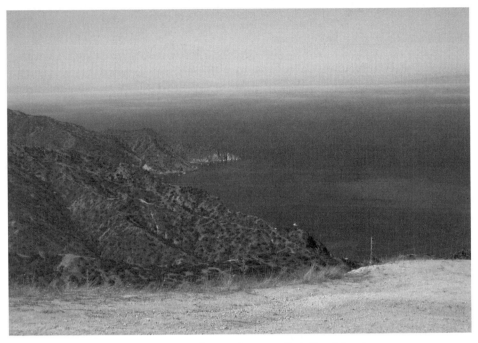

It's one postcard per minute at Catalina Island.

Description

Getting to the island is actually a lot of fun. A company called Catalina Express (**www.catalina express.com**) offers shuttle services from Downtown Long Beach Landing, Long Beach Queen Mary, Dana Point, and San Pedro; round-trip fares are reasonably priced at $56.50 plus a $6 bicycle fee. The boats are startlingly fast despite their immense size, so you'll reach the island in little more than one hour no matter which port you depart. Acquiring the passes is actually the only true hassle. Getting them requires you show up at the Conservancy office in Avalon with your bike and helmet during business hours with $20 and a credit card for the additional $40 deposit, refundable after returning the pass, which must be affixed to your handlebars in clear view.

After overcoming the bureaucratic hurdles, you're free to ride outside Avalon's city limits. Once you've navigated your way to the Hogsback Gate, you can begin the roughly 2-mile, 1,000-foot climb to East Summit. Keep an eye out for numerous shuttle vans and buses coming and going as you sweat your way to the top of the acacia-tree-lined roadway. Once you reach the top, you'll notice an overlook on the right that makes a great vantage point for peering across the San Pedro Channel to the bustling mainland you've escaped. Once you've taken in the panorama, continue on the paved road toward Catalina's own airstrip, dubbed "Airport in the Sky." Along the way, you can catch an eyeful of Catalina's steep coastline to your right and the long slopes and canyons that lead down to the western shores to your left. Since you've already handled the bulk of the ascent, the rest of the road is a rolling, flat affair, with no grinding climbs.

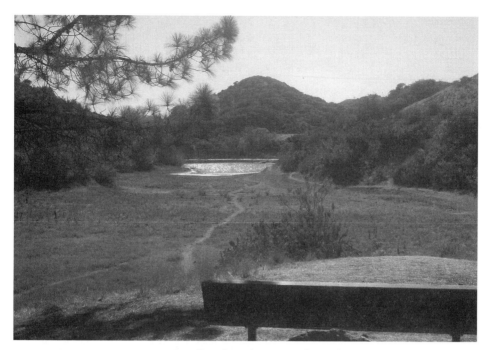

Yes, Catalina does have a real pond.

At roughly the 9.6-mile mark, you have the option of going to the diminutive Airport in the Sky to refill your water reserves and have a snack, which is not a bad idea since you have nearly 20 miles to go. After refueling, return to the road and turn right to begin your descent down the clearly marked Rancho Escondido Road. Resist the urge to go all out on this smooth, fast, groomed dirt road. Why? So you don't find yourself screeching to a halt amid a herd of startled American bison. Introduced to the island in 1924, these bison have thrived on the island since they were hunted to near extinction by American settlers in the 18th and 19th centuries. You will see them somewhere along the route, and although they are massive and look very intimidating, they will politely retreat as long as you approach them slowly.

At approximately the 13.3-mile mark, a relatively modern-looking horse ranch known as Rancho Escondido or Wrigley Ranch will come into view. Rumor has it that this site is still owned by the Wrigley family, who raise thoroughbred horses there. After passing by the ranch, hammer up a small climb, and then continue downhill toward Little Harbor.

Little Harbor will come into full view at about the 15-mile mark, where Rancho Escondido Road intersects Little Harbor Road. Turn left here, and head south along Cottonwood Beach, which could be a great place for a picnic and/or dip in the cool Pacific Ocean. After approximately 16.3 miles, traverse the cow crossing and make the short descent to the lower reaches of Middle Canyon on Middle Ranch Road.

The ascent up Middle Canyon on Middle Ranch Road is about 7 miles long, with a relatively easy grade that gains about 1,200 feet. Along the way, you'll see a very old building at about the 18.3-mile mark and a house with a large caged enclosure in front at roughly the 18.8-mile mark. Inside this cage, which you are welcome to view, is Tachi, a rare member of the island fox species. The fox is very small and tough to spot inside the spacious enclosure, but, because it's tame, it may come to find you first.

After visiting Tachi, continue up Middle Ranch Road. Just ahead lies Middle Ranch, which houses horses owned by residents of Avalon, as well as Catalina Island Conservancy employees.

Beyond Middle Ranch, the grade gets a little steeper before it terminates at its intersection with Airport Road, which you've already traveled. By now, you should be thoroughly bushed and severely saddle sore because you've ridden about 24 miles and conquered nearly 5,800 feet of climbing. Don't worry: relief is just under 5 mostly downhill miles away in Avalon, where you can ease the pain with ice cream (there's a parlor on nearly every corner), beer, and rich food. Unlike most of the other visitors and residents of the island, you've actually earned your indulgence.

After the Ride

The city of Avalon features a plethora of dining and drinking options within 1 square mile of its expanse. For great seafood, steaks, ribs, and a full bar with a New Orleans flair, stop by El Galleon on the beachfront, at 411 Crescent Avenue; (310) 510-1188. For breakfast on the water, look no farther than Antonio's Pizzeria and Cabaret, at 230 Crescent Avenue; (310) 510-0060.

33

CATALINA ISLAND: EAST END LOOP

KEY AT-A-GLANCE INFORMATION

Length: 12.75 miles

Configuration: Loop

Technical difficulty: 2

Aerobic difficulty: 4

Scenery: Casino Point, Abalone Point, Silver Canyon, Avalon Canyon, Avalon Bay, Pacific Ocean

Exposure: 100% exposed to sun

Trail traffic: Always light

Trail surface: Dry hardpack—no singletrack

Riding time: 2.5–3.5 hours

Access: Sunrise–sunset, 7 days

Maps: USGS 7.5-minute quad: Santa Catalina South

Special comments: A permit is required to pedal a bicycle anywhere outside Avalon's city limits. You can buy a permit from the Catalina Island Conservancy at the Conservancy House, 125 Claressa Avenue in Avalon, for $20, plus a $40 deposit that's refunded after the pass is returned; (310) 510-2595. Passes will not be issued if your bike doesn't have knobby tires or you don't have a helmet.

GPS TRAILHEAD COORDINATES (WGS84)

UTM Zone   11S
Easting   375833
Northing   3683422
Latitude   N 33.20'50"
Longitude   W 118.20'04"

In Brief

The East End Loop is the perfect introduction to mountain biking on Catalina Island. It features a priceless panorama of the city of Avalon, Avalon Canyon, Avalon Bay, and the East End, as well as some demanding climbing, for which the island is renowned. The route concludes with an exciting descent down Renton Mine Road, with fabulous views of the big, blue Pacific as a backdrop.

Safety Message

You have a very good chance of encountering bison on this route. For the most part, they are harmless—just approach them slowly and respectfully, and they will get out of your way.

Description

After resetting your odometer at Hogsback Gate, start ascending the paved hill to East Summit and Wrigley Reservoir. Keep an eye out for numerous shuttle vans and buses coming and going as you sweat your way to the top of the acacia-tree-lined roadway. You'll have sweated your way to East Summit at the 2-mile mark. After snapping some pictures at the overlook, turn back and head southward along the dirt road that runs along the east side of Wrigley Reservoir. Go around the left side of the gate to start your portage along the ridge on Divide Road.

DIRECTIONS

After arriving at Catalina Island by boat, helicopter, or plane, make your way to the north end of the oceanfront walk in Avalon, ride left up Marilla Avenue, and then turn right onto Vieudlou Avenue, followed by a left onto Stage Road. At the top of Stage Road, you will see a gate (Hogsback Gate) on your left; the route starts just beyond the gate.

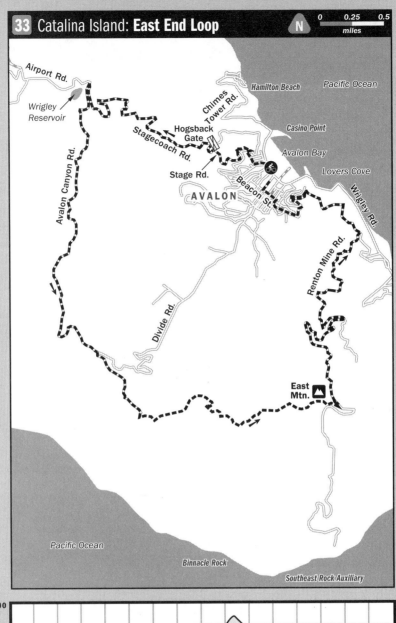

N

0   0.25   0.5
miles

Airport Rd.

Wrigley
Reservoir

Hamilton Beach   Pacific Ocean

Chimes Tower Rd.

Casino Point

Hogsback Gate

Stagecoach Rd.

Avalon Bay

Lovers Cove

Stage Rd.

Beacon St.

Wrigley Rd.

A V A L O N

Avalon Canyon Rd.

Renton Mine Rd.

Divide Rd.

East Mtn.

Pacific Ocean

Binnacle Rock

Southeast Rock Auxiliary

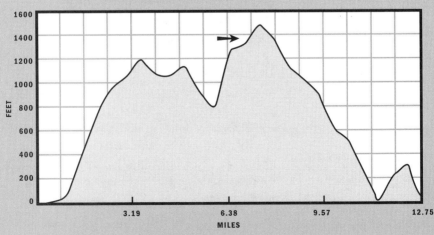

FEET				
1600				
1400				
1200				
1000				
800				
600				
400				
200				
0	3.19	6.38	9.57	12.75

MILES

Enjoy the views and pass one of the many trails that are off-limits to bikes at roughly the 4-mile mark, when you go by the intersection with Lone Tree Trail. A speedy descent ends at roughly the 4.9-mile mark, dumping you at the top of Avalon Canyon, where you'll pass the trail leading to Wrigley Botanical Garden—another trail you can't ride.

Continue beyond East Peak, visible on your right after a couple steep grinds, at roughly the 6.7-mile mark, and coast your way to East Mountain and another off-limits trail to East Mountain just beyond the 7.5-mile mark. Here you have a great view of the East End of Catalina Island. Ahead is a nearly 3-mile-long descent on Renton Mine Road that is by far the most fun downhill action found anywhere on the described routes, with plenty of smooth, fast turns to get sideways on.

Dirt gives way to pavement about 10.5 miles from Hogsback Gate, where a left turn takes you back into Avalon's city limits. Along the way, on the left, you can take a peep at The Inn at Mount Ada, a fancy hotel that was once William Wrigley Jr.'s private home.

If you haven't had enough of the Catalina Island mountain biking experience, give the Little Harbor Loop a shot. Despite much of Catalina's dirt roads being off-limits to bikes, it's still possible to ride all day on new terrain. Catalina's roads are wide, groomed, and user-friendly, and maps are available at the Conservancy for a modest $2. I hope someday the Conservancy will open up more terrain to mountain bikers. Until then, there are enough routes to make Catalina Island a legitimate fat-tire destination.

After the Ride

The city of Avalon features a plethora of dining and drinking options within 1 square mile of its expanse. For great seafood, steaks, ribs, and a full bar with a New Orleans flair, stop by El Galleon on the beachfront, at 411 Crescent Avenue; (310) 510-1188. For breakfast on the water, look no farther than Antonio's Pizzeria and Cabaret, at 230 Crescent Avenue; (310) 510-0060.

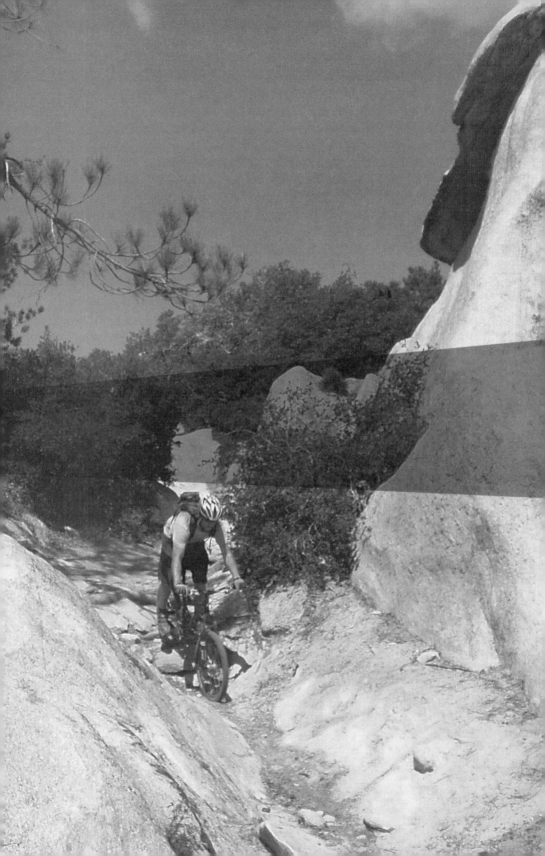

SOUTH BAY/CLEVELAND NATIONAL FOREST

EL MORO CANYON/ CRYSTAL COVE STATE PARK

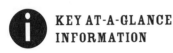

KEY AT-A-GLANCE INFORMATION

Length: 14.4 miles

Configuration: 2 loops

Technical difficulty: 3

Aerobic difficulty: 3

Scenery: Pacific Ocean

Exposure: 100% exposed to sunshine

Trail traffic: Moderate on weekdays, heavy on weekends

Trail surface: Dry hardpack with embedded rocks—15% singletrack

Riding time: 1.5–2.5 hours

Access: Sunrise–sunset, 7 days a week

Maps: USGS 7.5-minute quad: Laguna Beach

Special comments: Watch out for the numerous cactus plants that border upper sections of the trail.

In Brief

For all intents and purposes, this area can be referred to as "Sycamore Canyon Lite." It has all the environmental appeal of the Sycamore Canyon area of the northern Santa Monica Mountains, but in a more compact, manageable package. The described route is 14.4 miles and encompasses virtually all the terrain that Crystal Cove State Park has to offer. Minus the very technical, albeit short, descent on Redtail Ridge, all the other ascents and descents in the area are mellow and friendly. The trail maps posted on signs at virtually every intersection add to the area's cordiality. Although some maps are fading and difficult to read, they make the terrain very easy to navigate and have catchy names for each section of trail like "I Think I Can Hill" and "The Missing Link." All these elements create a vibe of user-friendliness that makes El Moro Canyon/Crystal Cove State Park a great place for newbie riders.

Description

Begin riding this abstract double-loop-shaped route on the unpaved "No Dogs" road, which originates at the paved road, northeast of the Crystal Cove State Park headquarters. After about 1.5 miles of mild climbing, turn right and descend "Mach One" Trail to its end at El Moro Canyon Trail. Turn right; then, after a slight, quarter-mile coast on El Moro Canyon Trail, turn left and start ascending "I Think I Can" Trail.

GPS TRAILHEAD COORDINATES (WGS84)

UTM Zone   11S
Easting   423729
Northing   3714404
Latitude   N 33.34'00"
Longitude   W 117.49'18"

DIRECTIONS

From Los Angeles, take Interstate 405 southbound to the CA 73 exit toward "San Diego Via Toll Road." Continue 5.76 miles on CA 73; then go south on CA 1 (Pacific Coast Highway) about 4 miles, and turn left into the entrance for El Moro Canyon/Crystal Cove State Park. The parking area and park facilities are less than a quarter mile up the driveway.

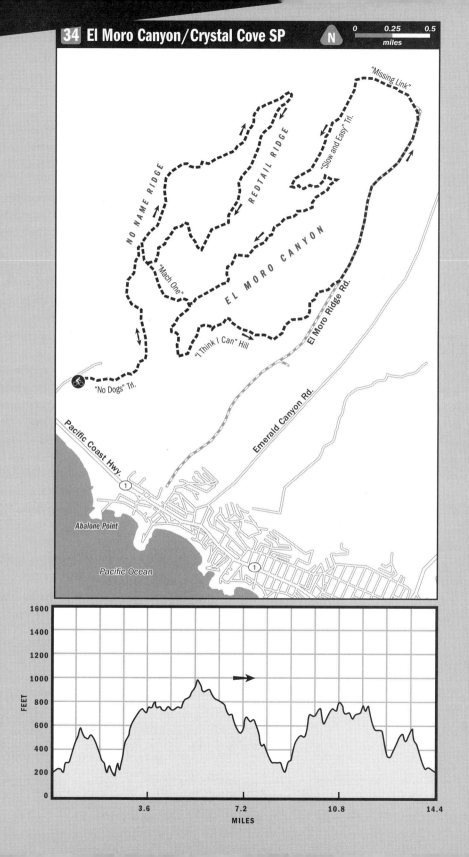

The name "I Think I Can" evokes images of something difficult, but in actuality the ascent is anything but. Roughly 600 feet of elevation are easily vanquished by the time you reach El Moro Ridge, at roughly the 3.7-mile mark, where you will turn left, heading northeast. After passing a campground and doing a little more easy climbing, turn left on the Missing Link singletrack, which should come into view on your left about 5.3 miles from the Crystal Cove State Park Headquarters. If you hit a gate, you've gone about a tenth of a mile too far on El Moro Ridge, so turn around and head back, keeping an eye out for a small trail offshoot on your right.

The roughly 0.6-mile-long foray on Missing Link is an exquisite singletrack experience, despite its low level of technical difficulty. Watch out for cacti, and turn left to descend Slow and Easy Trail for just over a mile back to El Moro Canyon Trail, marveling at how undeserving this mellow trail is of that safety-conscious moniker.

Hang a right at roughly the 7.2-mile mark, and continue descending on El Moro Canyon Trail back to "Mach One. Your casual, easy, "walk in the park" experience turns into minor masochism as you ascend the steepest continuous grade on this route on Mach One Trail. The pain continues after you turn right on No Name Ridge. Your next navigational objective requires making a right turn on an unnamed trail at about the 10-mile mark, allowing you to make a short descent followed by a short ascent to Redtail Ridge.

The most technically demanding portion of this route begins at roughly the 11-mile mark, where you turn right to descend the narrow Redtail Ridge singletrack. Things get really fun (or scary, depending on your technical prowess) when Redtail Ridge gets steeper at approximately 11.9 miles from the parking area. Lines will be tough to pick through this sandstone rock garden. Keep your weight back and your front end light so you don't endo on this section.

You're completely out of the danger zone at the 12.5-mile mark, where you'll follow the trail heading southwest as it returns, once again, to Mach One. Don't worry: you have to climb only the upper third of Mach One and your day's aerobic output is basically done.

After the Ride

For instant gratification, drive less than 3 miles north on CA 1 for a hearty deli sandwich made at lightning speed at Gallo's Italian Deli in Corona Del Mar, at 3900 East Coast Highway; (949) 675-7404. For fancier fare, drinks, and outdoor seating, visit Gulfstream Seafood, at 850 Avocado Avenue in nearby Newport Beach; (888) 243-4752.

35

KEY AT-A-GLANCE INFORMATION

Length: 7.5 miles

Configuration: Loop

Technical difficulty: 3

Aerobic difficulty: 3

Scenery: Jurupa Mountains, San Gabriel Mountains, San Bernardino Mountains

Exposure: 100% exposed to sunshine

Trail traffic: Light on weekdays, moderate on weekends

Trail surface: Dry hardpack with loose and embedded rocks, some sandy sections

Riding time: 1–2 hours

Access: Sunrise–sunset, 7 days a week

Maps: USGS 7.5-minute quad: Fontana

Special comments: If you attempt this ride in the summer, be prepared for the hottest temperatures in SoCal.

GPS TRAILHEAD COORDINATES (WGS84)

UTM Zone   11S

Easting   455352

Northing   3766684

Latitude   N 34.02'24"

Longitude   W 117.29'01"

FONTANA: JURUPA MOUNTAINS

In Brief

You may be wondering why anyone would have the audacity to recommend a mountain bike route that's smack in the middle of an urban wasteland—bordered on all sides by industry, traffic, pollution, and mass urban development. Because it's punk rock, that's why! The Jurupa Mountains offer an island oasis of natural beauty amid a concrete jungle. The single-track isn't too shabby out there either—amateur XC and downhill races (see **www.southridgeusa.com** for details) are regularly held there for that reason, and also because the Jurupa Mountains aren't governed by the same bureaucrats who have barred such events from happening everywhere else. You may want to get out there and enjoy the riding soon before the place gets permanently buried beneath factories and ugly tract housing.

Description

After hiding valuable belongings under your seats and locking your car, ride east across the empty dirt lot. Unless the bulldozers have been unleashed since this guide has been published, the lower end of a short mountain-cross course, complete with double jumps, should come into view. Pedal up the course in reverse, pondering what it would be like to clear the doubles on your ultra-light XC rig, if that's your mount of choice.

After realizing you're not Brian Lopes, continue beyond the course and ascend the trail that skirts the

DIRECTIONS

From Los Angeles, take Interstate 10 eastbound all the way to Fontana, and exit onto Cherry Avenue. Drive south on Cherry about 1.75 miles, and then turn left onto Live Oak Avenue. Southridge Park will appear immediately on your right; turn right into the driveway, and find a parking space in the lot.

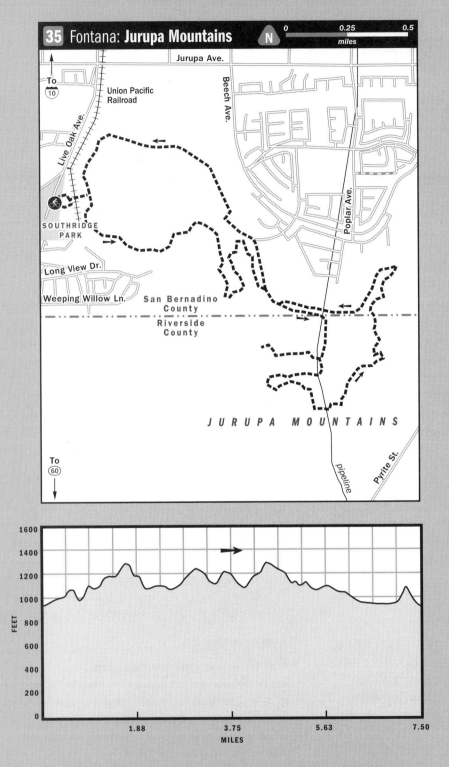

35 Fontana: **Jurupa Mountains**

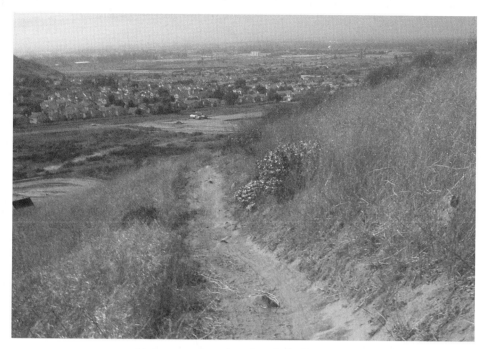

Nature meets urban jungle in Fontana.

hill to your left. After about a quarter mile, merge with the paved road and ascend to the water tanks at the end. Behind the tanks, the trail restarts and zigzags into the canyon below. At 2.5 miles, turn right into the canyon on a wide, sandy, dirt road. After roughly 0.3 miles on this road, ascend the singletrack on the right, heading west; it gets narrower and steeper as you go. The trail then loops around 180 degrees, and you'll be treated with a steep, rutted, at times sandy descent back to the canyon.

Next, cross the dirt road and cruise through the small grove of acacia trees, among which are the remnants of teenage debauchery, to the other side of the canyon, where another trail ascends the east side of the canyon. After a couple of switchbacks, the trail narrows to full singletrack and skirts the hillside heading north, ending at a dirt road where, at the 5-mile mark, you'll turn left and begin a portage bordering construction zones and drainage infrastructure. As you make your way back to your point of origin, keep an eye out for the road that leads back up to the water tanks; turn left here.

After about an eighth of a mile, a small singletrack that snakes back down northward to the drainage ditch will appear on your right. Turn left and ride the flood wash, following the road as it turns left to take you back to Southridge Park. If you've navigated properly, you'll be back at your car at roughly the 7-mile mark. If you're lucky enough, bureaucratic red tape and urban sprawl will have spared the racing events that are put on here by Southridge U.S.A., so you can come back another time and test your might against other riders in an XC race.

SAN JUAN TRAIL

KEY AT-A-GLANCE INFORMATION

Length: 8.7 miles

Configuration: Point-to-point shuttle run or out-and-back

Technical difficulty: 4

Aerobic difficulty: 2 for shuttle run, 4 for out-and-back

Scenery: Sugarloaf Peak, Cold Spring Canyon, Hot Spring Canyon, Lion Canyon, San Juan Canyon, Santa Ana Mountains

Exposure: 75% exposed to sun

Trail traffic: Light on weekdays, moderate on weekends

Trail surface: Dry hardpack with embedded rocks and roots—100% singletrack

Riding time: 2–3 hours

Access: Sunrise–sunset, 7 days a week

Maps: USGS 7.5-minute quads: Alberhill, Canada Gobernadora

Special comments: All parked vehicles must display Forest Adventure Passes, which you can purchase for $5 from various private vendors and ranger stations listed at www.fs.fed.us/r5/sanbernardino/ap/welcome.shtml.

GPS TRAILHEAD COORDINATES (WGS84)
(start of shuttle run)
UTM Zone 11S
Easting 458459
Northing 3723685
Latitude N 33.39'08"
Longitude W 117.26'53"

In Brief

The San Juan Trail truly is one of the finest stretches of singletrack in SoCal. The trail boasts every feature of an ideal two-wheeled romp, including technical rock gardens, steep bomb runs, kickers, and fast-banked turns, with the picturesque panorama of the Santa Ana Mountains in the Cleveland National Forest as an exquisite backdrop. Switchbacks form the defining characteristic of this playground: more are found on this 8.7-mile stretch than in any other locale—I lost count after ten in the first mile of ascent. Although this ride is recommended as a shuttle run, it is probably best enjoyed ridden up and then down. The throbbing pain in your legs and lungs is hard to notice when there is so much to see and so many obstacles to negotiate. If your bike was built for anything other than downhill duty and you've got the time, please abort the shuttling mission. Better yet, ride the whole thing and then shuttle it, because afterward you'll surely want another slice of downhill indulgence.

Description

Since you're entering remote territory, prepare for this ride as you would for any cross-country epic, with air,

DIRECTIONS

From Los Angeles, take I-405 south to San Juan Capistrano, and exit at CA 74 (Ortega Highway). Head north on CA 74 about 12.5 miles, and turn left at the San Juan Fire Station. Drive past the fire station, and continue about 0.75 miles until you reach the dirt lot, bathroom, and signs for San Juan Trail. Stage one of your vehicles here if you're shuttling; load bikes, gear, and people into a second vehicle, and return to CA 74; head north about 9.2 miles, turn left onto Long Canyon Road, and, after about 2.5 miles, park on the left in front of the upper entrance to San Juan Trail. Blue Jay Campground sits just beyond the entrance.

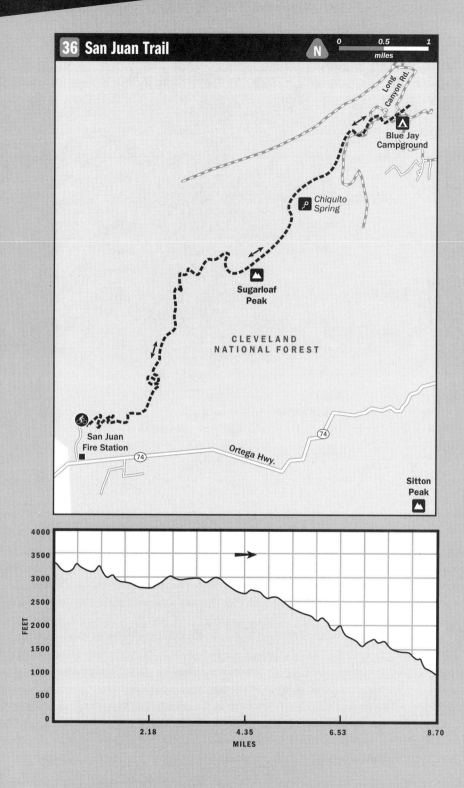

N

0   0.5   1
miles

Long Canyon Rd

Blue Jay
Campground

Chiquito
Spring

Sugarloaf
Peak

CLEVELAND
NATIONAL FOREST

San Juan
Fire Station

74

Ortega Hwy.

74

Sitton
Peak

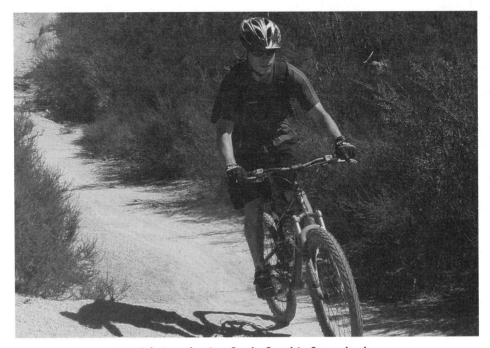

Patrick Rose having fun before his frame broke

tubes, jacket, snacks, tools, maximum water, and a cell phone, if possible. You may be wondering why a shuttle run requires all the gear. You need all that stuff because you simply never know what is going to happen. My riding buddy had a frame failure smack-dab in the middle of the route. An incident like that usually results in a lot of hiking (that's where the water and snacks come in handy) if the frame cannot be fixed (tools) and the rider wasn't injured (cell phone).

The route starts with an oak-shaded descent that is particularly steep and technical because of large embedded rocks and deep rain ruts. At about 1.5 miles, continue straight at the intersection, following the path most traveled. After the intersection, the trail flattens out as you pass under tall oaks. At about 2 miles, dismount for a creek crossing atop a sketchy natural bridge made of oak tree roots. After the crossing, ascend a short but steep and technical climb, which presents a challenge rarely encountered anywhere in SoCal—tree roots, lots of them.

After the root-addled ascent, you'll see no major elevation gains or losses, but the terrain will morph from shaded oak forest floor to a manzanita grove with orange-hued soil fully exposed to sunshine. At the 3.5-mile mark, after you pass the rocky Sugarloaf Peak on your right, the trail turns sharply to the right (ignore the narrow trail going left) and becomes rocky and technical for the next half mile. After the rocky sections, the trail levels out and becomes the archetypal singletrack for which it is famous—narrow, fast, unimpeded by foliage, with sweeping, bermed corners, and composed of a grippy, dry, compact, orange crust. The waist-level manzanita plants that dominate the area aren't tall enough to block your view of approaching corners, but don't lean into them—the stems are less forgiving than steel wire and will rip you off your bike. You'll have several opportunities to lose contact with the ground in this section for some hang time, but it's up to you to find the right line that leads to the kicker.

After the 6-mile mark, the trail gets looser and steeper, with a series of somewhat challenging turns and switchbacks. Get used to turning because at about the 8.4-mile mark, you'll have to negotiate ten-plus very tight switchbacks before you get dumped out into the lower parking lot at roughly 8.7 miles, marking the end of your ride.

GPS Trailhead Coordinates (WGS84)

(End of shuttle run)
UTM Zone 11S
Easting 452589
Northing 3718052
Latitude N 33.36'04"
Longitude W 117.30'40"

After the Ride

The immediate vicinity of San Juan Trail offers zero food-serving venues, so your best bet for immediate nourishment after the ride is to bring your own. If you left your cooler at home and are sick of energy goo, try dining at former president Richard Nixon's favorite Mexican restaurant, El Adobe de Capistrano, at 31891 Camino Capistrano in San Juan Capistrano; (949) 493-1163. For cheaper but by no means less presidential Mexican cuisine, stop by Las Golondrinas, at 27124 Paseo Espada, Suite 803; (949) 240-3440.

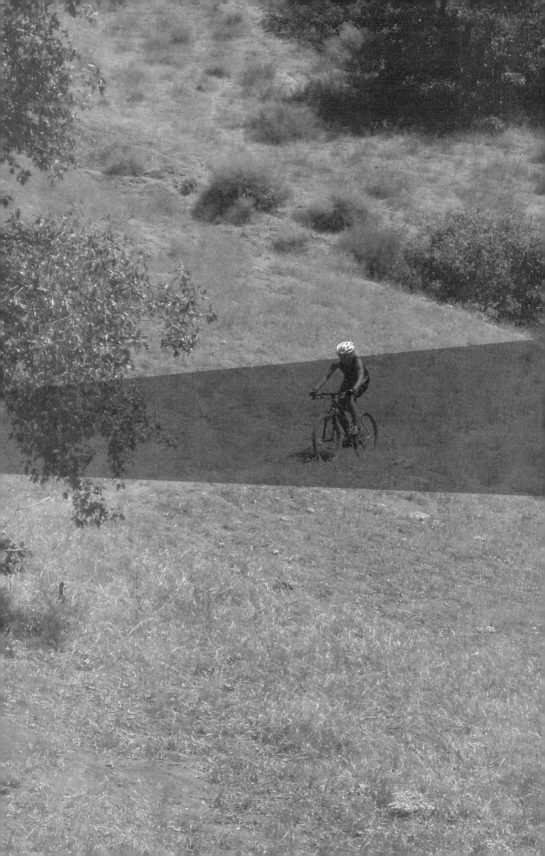

BEYOND LOS ANGELES COUNTY

LOWER ROCK CREEK TRAIL

KEY AT-A-GLANCE INFORMATION

Length: 7.8 miles

Configuration: Point-to-point shuttle ride

Technical difficulty: 5

Aerobic difficulty: 1

Scenery: Lower Rock Creek Canyon

Exposure: 30% exposed to sunshine

Trail traffic: Light–moderate on weekdays, moderate–heavy on weekends

Trail surface: Varies from loose and rocky to sandy and loamy—95% singletrack

Riding time: 0.5–1.5 hours

Access: Sunrise–sunset, 7 days a week

Maps: USGS 7.5-minute quad: Casa Diablo Mountain, Tom's Place, Rovana

Special comments: Sharp-edged rocks are common on this route, so be prepared with a spare tube, tire levers, a patch kit, and a source of air.

GPS TRAILHEAD COORDINATES (WGS84)

UTM Zone 11S
Easting 353400
Northing 4157965
Latitude N 37.33'25"
Longitude W 118.39'35"

In Brief

Any complaints about the 286-mile drive to get here will be quashed by one shuttle run down Lower Rock Creek Trail. This route involves a beautifully crafted singletrack that parallels Rock Creek as it cascades through a massive gorge of its own making, dropping nearly 2,000 feet from Tom's Place to the Owens Valley floor. The lower half of the trail is very technical and can be ridden completely dab-free by only the best riders on the planet. You'll find lots of great places to picnic and swim on the way down. With no admission fee, Lower Rock Creek Trail is definitely a great alternative to bombing the downhill runs at Mammoth Mountain.

Description

Once you've gotten all your cars and riders properly situated, start your bomb down the trail, but don't forget one

DIRECTIONS

From Los Angeles, take Interstate 405 north to I-5 north; go 3.1 miles, and join CA 14, driving 118.3 miles until it becomes US 395. Continue 122 miles on US 395 to the town of Bishop. Drive 12 miles beyond the US 395–US 6 junction, on US 395, until you reach an exit for Gorge Road. Turn left onto Gorge Road, and then right onto Lower Rock Creek Road after about 0.2 miles. Continue up Lower Rock Creek Road about 3 miles until it crosses Lower Rock Creek and makes a 180-degree turn. Here, you'll see the site of a former campground and restaurant. Leave one vehicle here, load the bikes and riders in a second vehicle, and continue up Lower Rock Creek Road about 7.9 miles (it actually becomes Old Sherwin Grade Road along the way) until it rejoins US 395. The upper entrance to Lower Rock Creek Trail is just before the intersection with US 395 and is clearly marked by a sign. Park opposite the trail entrance, along Old Sherwin Grade Road.

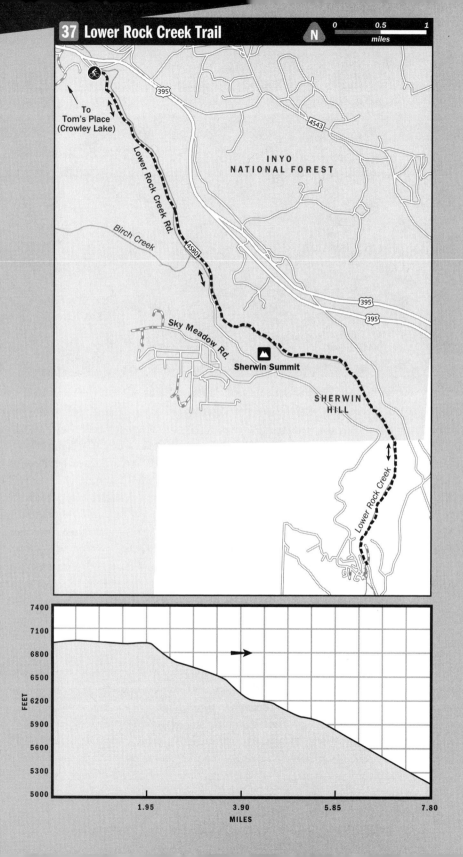

To
Tom's Place
(Crowley Lake)

395

4543

INYO
NATIONAL FOREST

Lower Rock Creek Rd.

Birch Creek

4S80

Sky Meadow Rd.

Sherwin Summit

395

395

SHERWIN
HILL

Lower Rock Creek

7400
7100
6800
6500
6200
5900
5600
5300
5000

FEET

1.95   3.90   5.85   7.80

MILES

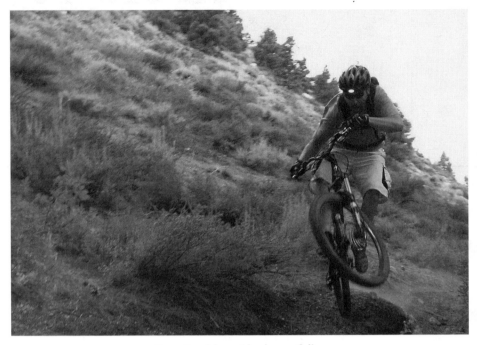

Keep it rubber-side down, folks.

very important item—the keys to the vehicle at the bottom. Without these, you'll have to lug your heavy downhill rigs up Lower Rock Creek Road, which is an excruciating grinder.

For the first 2 miles of the ride, you'll need to pedal hard to get any speed because you'll lose relatively little elevation over that stretch. Nevertheless, a few fast sections will give you an idea of what this trail is about—a pristine foot-wide path of varying soil compositions that often snakes among trees, giving the rider three dimensions of technical riddles to solve. The soil on the first section is the driest on the route, with far fewer rocks than down below. Things don't get really interesting until after the first road crossing.

The trail dumps you out onto Sherwin Grade Road roughly 2.1 miles from the start. After looking for fast-moving traffic, ride up the road a few feet (north), and look for the reentry to the trail on the other side. The trail immediately gets exciting. Watch out for a nice little kicker on the right side about a quarter of a mile in. Much of this section is composed of both wet and dry loam, but it still doesn't deliver any hurdles of great technical difficulty. After roughly 1 mile, you'll cross the road one last time.

The entrance is easily visible directly across the road. At this entry, the trail becomes a steep chute, diverging from the road completely. At about 3.8 miles from the start, a wood bridge takes you to the north side of the creek, and the trail morphs into a rocky mess. The remaining 4 miles are action-packed—very rocky and technical—difficult to clean on even a 10-inch travel-downhill rig. About halfway through this section, the trail flattens out a bit, and you'll see several snack and rest areas among the tall pines. Take a break, and take in your surroundings—you're inside the trough of a deep gorge carved through dense granite

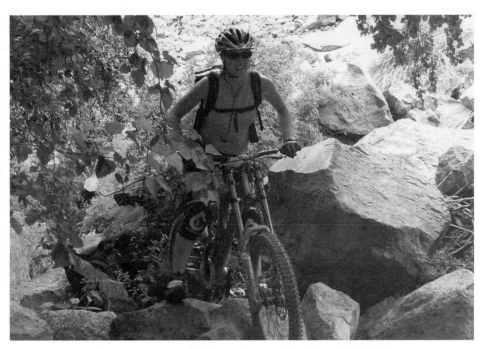

On her next run, Gabriela rode over this obstacle dab-free.

over thousands of years. The trail is the only way out, which is fine, provided your body or bike didn't sustain any damage on the way down.

To cool off, take a dip in the snowmelt runoff that is Lower Rock Creek—after all, you've been cooking in 90-plus-degree heat—then hop back on your rig and finish the descent. You will most certainly need to do another run. A mere 7.8 miles of singletrack of this caliber isn't enough to justify the long drive out here. No matter how many runs you take, you can laugh at the masses that flocked to Mammoth Ski Resort and forked over large dough to ride the dusty, pumice-covered turf there. For merely the cost of gas, you probably had more fun than they did.

After the Ride

For tasty burgers and suds, visit Tom's Place Café, at 8189 Crowley Lake Drive in the town of Crowley Lake; (760) 935-4239. For bonehead mistakes like leaving your helmet or cycle shoes at home—300 miles from the trail—Aerohead Cycles in Bishop can get you outfitted. They are at 312 North Warren Street; (760) 873-4151.

38

MOVIE ROAD LOOP

KEY AT-A-GLANCE INFORMATION

Length: 17.5 miles

Configuration: Loop

Technical difficulty: 2

Aerobic difficulty: 4

Scenery: Mount Whitney, Mount Langley, Mount Williamson, Inyo Mountains, Alabama Hills

Exposure: 100% exposed to sunshine

Trail traffic: Very light

Trail surface: Pavement and washboarded fire roads with sandy sections—no singletrack

Riding time: 2.5–3.5 hours

Access: Sunrise–sunset, 7 days a week

Maps: USGS 7.5-minute quad: Mount Langley, Manzanar, Lone Pine

Special comments: The potential heat, coupled with high altitude, can make this an exhausting ride, so bring plenty of water. Be wary of speeding cars on Whitney Portal Road.

GPS TRAILHEAD COORDINATES (WGS84)
UTM Zone   11S
Easting   400736
Northing   4050641
Latitude   N 36°35'46"
Longitude   W 118°06'35"

In Brief

Driving 200 miles to do a bike ride only makes sense if the route is extraordinary. The Movie Road Loop, though it lacks technical difficulty, presents a 360-degree view of the towering Mount Whitney and picturesque Alabama Hills that will leave you in awe. In fact, the views are so spectacular that hundreds of Hollywood movies have been filmed here over the years.

Description

Once you've parked your vehicle and completed your pre-ride prep and rituals, start pedaling up Whitney Portal Road. Before you get out the saddle and start hammering, keep in mind that the scale here is distorted by the massive peaks in the distance and the clear mountain air. The base of the mountains, your destination, actually lies almost 6 miles ahead, though it may look like 1 or 2 miles at most. Pace yourself and get into a nice groove because you will ascend more than 2,000 feet over that stretch, and the air just gets thinner and thinner as you go.

The staggeringly beautiful mountains up ahead offer a nice distraction from the pain that may be building in your lungs, heart, and legs. You're looking at three separate peaks of more than 14,000 feet: Mount Langley, ahead and left, reaches 14,027 feet; Mount Whitney, directly ahead, ranks as the highest in the continental

DIRECTIONS

From Los Angeles, take I-405 north to I-5 north. Continue 3.1 miles on I-5 north, and then join CA 14; continue northbound 118.3 miles until I-5 becomes US 395. After 64.5 miles, turn left onto Whitney Portal Road, right in the middle of downtown Lone Pine. Continue another 2.75 miles, and park at the intersection of Movie Road and Whitney Portal Road, which is clearly marked by a sign.

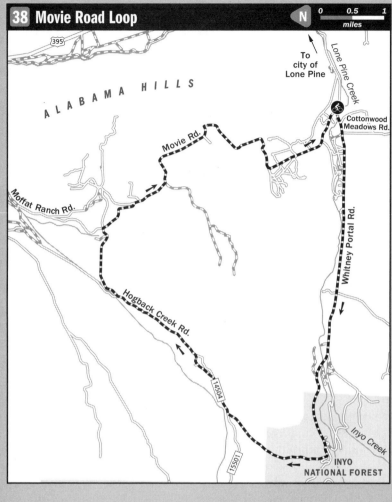

N

0   0.5   1
miles

395

A L A B A M A   H I L L S

To
city of
Lone Pine

Lone Pine Creek

Movie Rd.

Cottonwood
Meadows Rd.

Moffat Ranch Rd.

Whitney Portal Rd.

Hogback Creek Rd.

14S04

15S01

Inyo Creek

INYO
NATIONAL FOREST

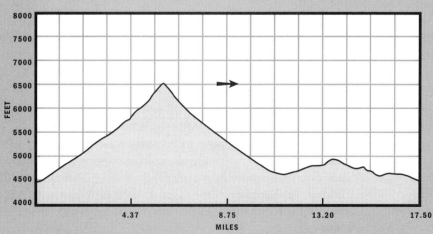

8000
7500
7000
6500
6000
5500
5000
4500
4000

FEET

4.37   8.75   13.20   17.50
MILES

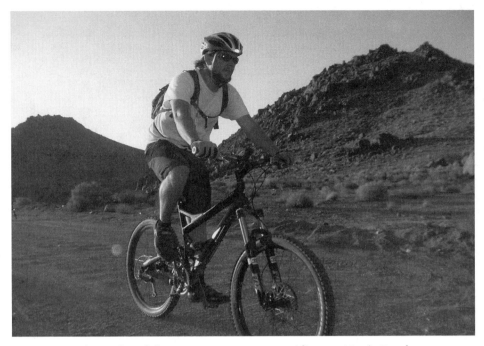

The author doing some extreme stunt riding on Movie Road

United States at 14,494 feet; and to the right stands Mount Williamson, reaching 14,375 feet above sea level.

When you do reach the right turn for Hogback Creek Road, about 5.9 miles from your car, you'll be directly at the base of the aforementioned peaks. For those daring enough, continue the rest of the grind up Whitney Portal Road to gain an additional more than 2,000 feet of elevation over about half the distance (3 miles). If you make it, you'll be rewarded with a picnic area for lounging, big trees, and views of Lone Pine Creek cascading down from the heavens.

Mere mortals should avoid serious pain and turn right at Hogback Creek Road, which is signposted. The first 2 miles of this fire road are wide, groomed, and steep, making it the perfect place to break your previous top-speed record. After that, the road starts to flatten out. Sand and washboarding provide the only technical challenges on this stretch, and for the rest of the route. To deal with either subtlety, just look for the flattest, most compact part of the road, which can usually be found in the middle or on the sides. None of the sand is so deep that you'll have to stop and walk, but it can get sketchy and cumbersome.

At roughly 11.6 miles from the start, just after the slight grade of Hogback Road ends and you start to climb again, make a right onto Movie Road, which will be marked with a large sign. The next 2 miles comprise a relaxing climb into the heart of the Alabama Hills—a VW-sized, granite-boulder-strewn desert area. It's obvious why this area has been featured in numerous Hollywood films—*Tremors*, starring Kevin Bacon, may come to mind—it's an idyllic Old West setting, with tumbleweeds in the foreground and towering gold-concealing peaks on the horizon.

If you've timed your departure right, the sun should be setting as you spin your way across the final 3 miles. Unless you stared at the ground for the entire ride, you'll be moved to tears the beauty of the Movie Road Loop, and you may have a new view on cycling in general. Mountain biking isn't always about hang time and adrenaline; it's about getting in touch with nature—and the route you just completed is proof.

After the Ride

For a complete Movie Road experience, replenish your spent calories in Lone Pine at the Mount Whitney Restaurant, at 227 South Main Street, and treat yourself to great diner food while admiring decor that pays homage to Lone Pine's extensive history as a film location; (760) 876-5751.

39

GRIDLEY/PRATT/ COZY DELL LOOP

Length: 22.8 miles

Configuration: Loop

Technical difficulty: 4

Aerobic difficulty: 5

Scenery: Ojai Valley, Gridley Canyon, Nordhoff Peak, Nordhoff Ridge, Stewart Canyon, Pacific Ocean, Lake Casitas, Ventura County, Channel Islands

Exposure: 70% exposed to sunshine

Trail traffic: Light on weekdays, moderate on weekends

Trail surface: Mostly hardpack, with embedded rocks and some loose, shaley sections—55% singletrack

Riding time: 4–6 hours

Access: Sunrise–sunset, 7 days a week

Maps: USGS 7.5-minute quads: Matilija, Ojai, Lion Canyon

Special comments: Because of the huge amount of climbing involved, bring at least 70 ounces of water and some snacks.

GPS TRAILHEAD
COORDINATES (WGS84)
UTM Zone 11S
Easting 293314
Northing 3815515
Latitude N 34.27'38"
Longitude W 119.15'00"

In Brief

With more than 5,000 feet of total elevation gain, the Gridley/Pratt/Cozy Dell Loop is a true ass-kicker. Don't let its measly 22-plus miles fool you—the first 11 miles are mostly uphill, and the climbing just increases in severity the farther you go. The last 0.75 miles are devastatingly steep, but your effort will be rewarded with one of the best panoramic views anywhere. The downhill is just as intense, with plenty of off-camber turns and embedded rocks to enrich your endorphins. This route is perhaps the most challenging single loop in SoCal. Prepare to be humbled, no matter how in shape you think you are.

Description

Because you're about to embark on one of the most physically demanding rides of your life, you may want to extend your normal pre-ride prep to include rituals like contacting dead relatives, transcendental meditation, yoga, and possibly Pilates. At the very least, stretch a little, fill your H_2O receptacles to the brim, and pack two tubes, a patch kit, a multitool, a cell phone, and snacks. This ride is so demanding that you'll definitely need calorie replenishment at some point during the climb. Something that's easy on your stomach will work best: an energy drink, carbohydrate goo, or some other liquid supplement.

  After you've made peace with your deity of choice, hop on your steed and start climbing Pratt Trail. The first 1.5 miles of Pratt are a rock garden, so unless you have

DIRECTIONS

From Los Angeles, take US 101 north about 50 miles; then take the CA 33 exit north toward Ojai. After about 13.2 miles, merge with CA 150 east; turn left onto Signal Street after 1 mile. Continue on Signal about 1 mile until it terminates in a dirt lot. Park here and find the trailhead at the southwest end of the lot.

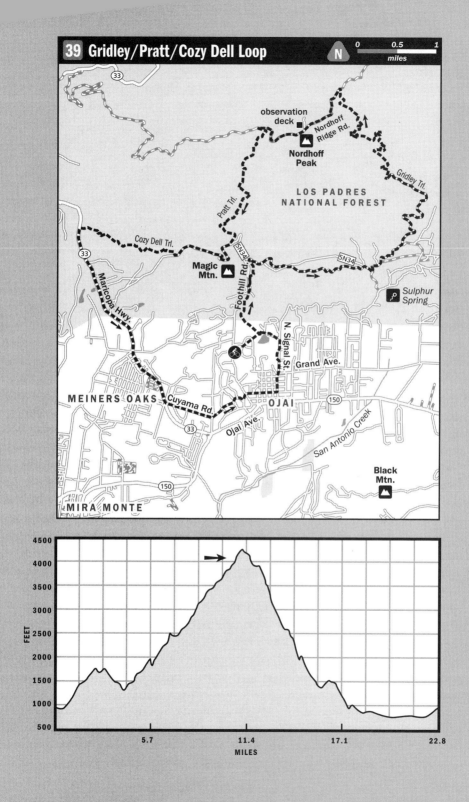

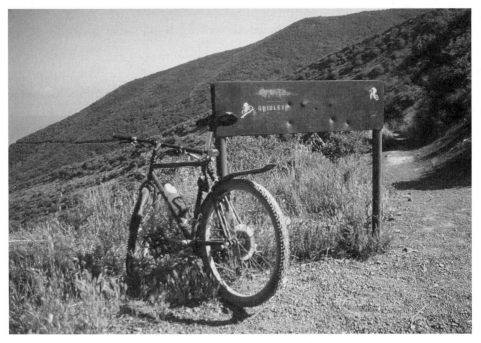

Mike Stanosek's bike at the top of Gridley

uncanny trail bike skills, you'll be carrying your ride over much of it. This section of trail is unique because it skirts the boundaries of several parcels of private land, and at one point you're literally in someone's backyard.

Leave Pratt Trail for later by turning right onto the fire road at roughly 1.8 miles from the start. This road begins as a wide, groomed fire road but becomes singletrack about half-way along as it traverses over to Gridley Trail for just over 2 miles. Although this is a traverse, it still involves a healthy dose of climbing. You'll know you're at Gridley when you see an avocado grove—at this point, roughly 4 miles from the start, turn left and start ascending the fire road that rises through the avocado-covered hillside.

Provided you haven't stopped to make guacamole, continue beyond the grove and start Gridley Trail proper, which is the prototypical SoCal singletrack—narrow, dry hardpack with embedded sandstone rocks scented by the fragrant flora of the chaparral environment. The route doesn't get really steep and hairy until just beyond the 7-mile mark, when a mellow trail of mild grade becomes a steep, seemingly never-ending series of switchbacks and false summits that will have you begging for mercy. The Gridley singletrack comes to an end at Nordhoff Fire Road, roughly 9.7 miles from the start. Most bikers get to relax here because attempting the remaining grind to Nordhoff Peak would be insanity.

Since you're living on the edge on this particular day, put away your camera and snacks and hang a left onto Nordhoff Road to crest the summit. Even if you hadn't just completed one of the hardest singletrack ascents in SoCal, this last climb would be brutal because, although it's groomed and flat, Nordhoff Road is very steep. Huff and puff your way to the top. At roughly the 11-mile mark, a short spur of road climbs the hill to the right to a large steel observatory. Please check it out! It's definitely worth the extra pain. On a clear day, you can see the Channel Islands from there.

After enjoying the panorama, head back to Nordhoff Road, continue westbound about 0.8 miles, and turn left onto Pratt Trail, which is marked by a sign that has an arrow and the words SIGNAL ROAD: 5 MILES. Signal Road is where you parked your car, remember? Turn left here and begin the descent of nasty, narrow Pratt Trail. The main hazard on this trail is not an overwhelming number of rocks but many off-camber turns and areas where it's very easy to slide off the trail. Provided your tires aren't overinflated and your knobbies are fresh, this section should not be a problem if you're wary and skilled.

At about 14.6 miles from the start, Pratt Trail will reach a junction with Cozy Dell Fire Road. Turn right here, and continue about 1.1 miles until you reach a singletrack that branches off to the right—this is Cozy Dell Trail—for the last chapter in this saga. If you're not so thoroughly thrashed that you can ride this 2-mile stretch of rock gardens and switchbacks without collapsing in the bushes or crashing, you're definitely in good shape. At 17.7 miles, turn left onto CA 33 to conclude your route on pavement. Just beyond the 20.2-mile mark, turn left onto Cuyama Road, and stay on Cuyama until it becomes East Aliso Street. Turn left onto Signal Street to return to your car.

Congratulations: you've just completed one of the nastiest rides in SoCal! The only route that rivals this one in terms of elevation gain is the Mount Wilson Toll Road, but this route is arguably much tougher because much of the climbing takes place on technical singletrack that keeps you out of the saddle most of the time. Consider the Gridley/Pratt/Cozy Dell Loop a right of passage, making you a fat-tire crusader of the highest order.

After the Ride

After so many hours in the bush, it totally makes sense to dine on wild game and wash it down with Guinness on tap at The Deer Lodge in Ojai, at 2261 Maricopa Highway; (805) 646-4256. For more-immediate gratification, try Oh Hi Frostie for burgers and milkshakes, at 214 West Ojai Avenue; (805) 646-1923.

MOUNT PINOS/ McGILL TRAIL

KEY AT-A-GLANCE INFORMATION

Length: 13.25 miles

Configuration: Point-to-point shuttle run

Technical difficulty: 4

Aerobic difficulty: 3

Scenery: Mount Pinos, Los Padres National Forest, Cuddy Valley

Exposure: Mostly shaded by tall pine trees

Trail traffic: Light on weekdays, moderate–heavy on weekends

Trail surface: Varies from dry hard-pack, to hard-packed loam with some loose, rocky areas—100% singletrack

Riding time: 1–2 hours

Access: Sunrise–sunset, 7 days a week

Maps: USGS 7.5-minute quads: Sawmill Mountain, Cuddy Valley

Special comments: Be prepared for mechanical failures (bring spare tubes and patch kits) and for high-speed crashes (pack first-aid supplies). Snow and ice can be present in the fall and early spring.

GPS TRAILHEAD COORDINATES (WGS84)

UTM Zone 11S
Easting 309177
Northing 3856626
Latitude N 34.50'03"
Longitude W 119.05'12"

In Brief

Although this route can be ridden continuously as an out-and-back or as an obscured figure-eight, it is best enjoyed as a shuttle run for downhill enthusiasts. This way you can use a downhill or freeride bike outside the confines of a ski resort. The route can, however, be enjoyed by any discipline of two-wheeled locomotion, and it offers a forested, high-altitude riding experience otherwise unavailable so close to LA County.

Description

Remember that scene in *Star Wars Episode VI: Return of the Jedi* when Luke Skywalker engaged two storm troopers in a high-speed chase on hovering motorcycles on the forest moon of Endor? Descending Mount Pinos is somewhat like that, but without fuzzy Ewoks and Darth Vader's army chasing you. In short, it is possibly one of the most exhilarating descents in California.

If you aren't of the school of thought that insists every descent is a reward to be enjoyed only after a long, grueling ascent, you'll find shuttling this ride advantageous for two reasons: 1) The pavement climb up Mount Pinos Road (Forest Service Road 9N04) is a snoozer and can be hot and buggy to boot. 2) Ascending McGill Trail is absolutely grueling on a long-travel rig. Save your energy for the descent.

DIRECTIONS

From Los Angeles, take I-405 north toward Sacramento until it becomes I-5 north. Stay on I-5 46.1 miles, and exit onto Frazier Mountain Park Road. Turn left, and after 6 miles, bear right on Cuddy Valley Road to reach Lockwood Valley Road. Continue 6 miles to Mount Pinos Highway, and then continue another 5 miles to McGill Campground, where you will park.

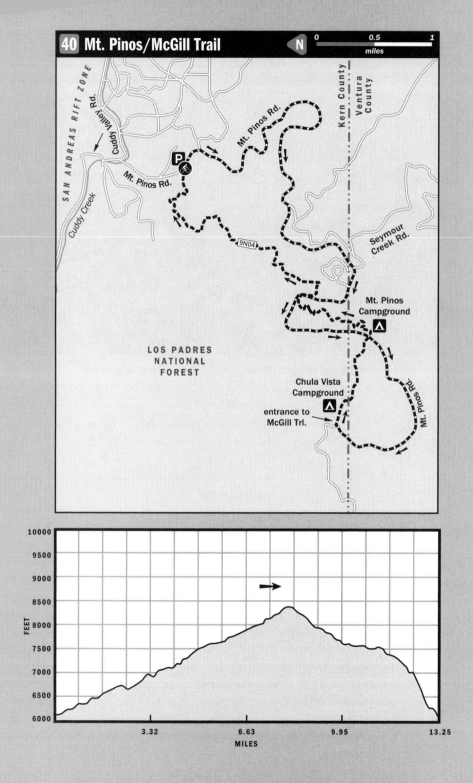

40 Mt. Pinos/McGill Trail

N

0   0.5   1
miles

SAN ANDREAS RIFT ZONE

Cuddy Valley Rd.

Mt. Pinos Rd.

P

Mt. Pinos Rd.

Cuddy Creek

Mt. Pinos Rd.

Kern County
Ventura County

9N04

Seymour Creek Rd.

Mt. Pinos Campground

LOS PADRES NATIONAL FOREST

Chula Vista Campground

entrance to McGill Trl.

Mt. Pinos Rd.

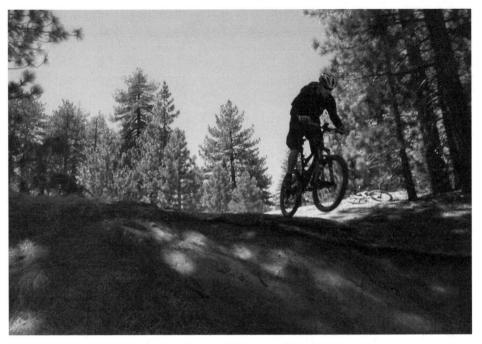

Mount Pinos is a real blast, and it's shady too.

Park one vehicle at the bottom of McGill Trail where it intersects with Mount Pinos Highway, and drive the other, loaded with bikes and passengers, up the road 8.4 miles until it ends at Chula Vista Campground. Before you start the descent, you may want to take a little ride to the summit of Mount Pinos, just to say you did it. It's only a 2.6-mile out-and-back. Originating from the start of the driveway to Chula Vista Campground, it includes a paltry 500-foot elevation gain to get your legs warm.

Your descent begins at the southeast end of the Chula Vista parking lot, just to the right of the ranger's cabin, if you're facing east. A couple of picnic areas will appear on your left in the first mile. Just follow the tire tracks and stay to the right. Bomb down the hill, staying wary of roots, ruts, and loose rocks. After roughly 1 mile, you'll cross Mount Pinos Road and see an elementary drop at the crest of a small hillside. Catch some air, and continue down the trail. Roughly an eighth of a mile after the road crossing, traverse Mount Pinos Campground in a straight line and rejoin the trail on the north side. Testing your airborne composure will be the theme of the next 1.2 miles, as there are several water-bar jumps in the trail. If you're new to jumping, just slow down and roll them. If you hit them at a higher speed, commit, pull upward, and don't panic-brake at the last second or you will endo.

Roughly 2.4 miles from the Chula Vista parking lot, hang a right onto Mount Pinos Road and then rejoin the trail on the left after about 200 feet of tarmac. The next 2.6 miles evoke the aforementioned visions of *Return of the Jedi*. There is a little climbing and a few flat sections in the first mile, but after that you'll move about 1,250 feet closer to sea level in just 1.6 miles at a blistering pace. This is primo singletrack because of its narrowness, soil composition, and forested scenery. Ample traction is provided by the decaying pine needles that blanket the forest floor, trapping precious bits of moisture. There are no drops or water bars to jump here, but the narrow straightaways, sweeping turns, and mild switchbacks will easily get your adrenaline going. If you see a hiker, horseback rider, or ascending mountain biker, slow down, yield the right-of-way and cheerfully inform him or her how many riders are behind you.

After carving your way back to your car, shuttle it again! Pedaling purists get only one shot at the descent, unless they are training for La Ruta de los Conquistadores (an epic 100-mile race in Costa Rica) and plan to repeat the entire route a second time. Shoot, Mount Pinos is so much fun, you may want to do it a third time.

After the Ride

Dining options are few and far between out here in the sticks, so your best bet is to bring your own food and beverages. If you brought no table fare, go to the Mountain View Mini Mart, at 6929 Lockwood Valley Road in Frazier Park, for splendid deli sandwiches and bottled drinks; (661) 245-1653.

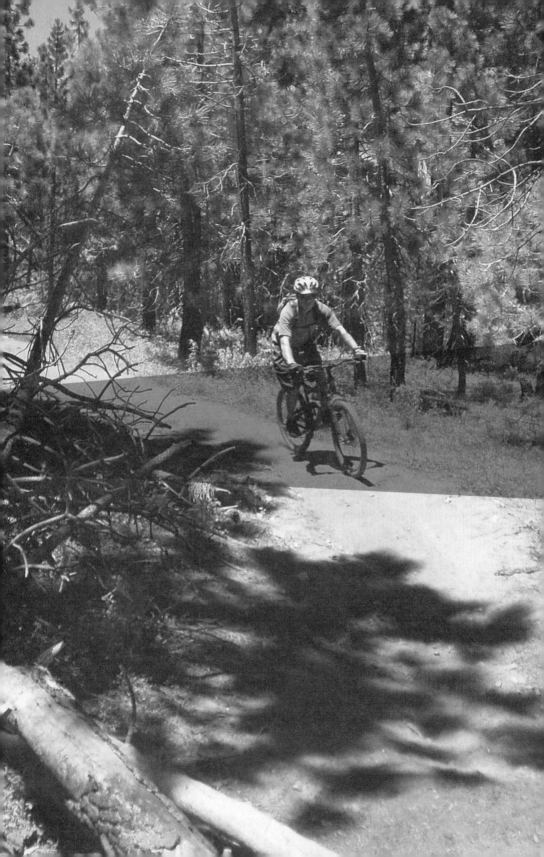

APPENDIXES AND INDEX

Appendix A: Don't leave home without . . .

Bicycle multitool
Bike pump or CO_2 system (three cartridges per rider)
Cell phone
Chain lube
Chain tool, plus small extra length of chain and three pins
First-aid kit
Maps and/or GPS unit
Nutrition bars and/or energy goo
One extra tire
100 ounces of water per rider
One or more riding buddies and a positive attitude
Patch kit (if using tubeless tires, make sure you have a tubeless kit)
Sunblock
Two spare tubes per rider
Tire leavers

Appendix B: If you feel like giving back to your sport . . .

CORBA (Concerned Off-Road Bicyclists Association)
www.corbamtb.com
P.O. Box 575576
Sherman Oaks, CA 91413
(818) 773-3555

IMBA (International Mountain Bike Association)
www.imba.com
P.O. Box 7578
Boulder, CO 80306
(888) 442-4622

LACBC (Los Angeles County Bicycle Coalition)
www.labikecoalition.org
634 South Spring Street, Suite 821
Los Angeles, CA 90014
(213) 629-2142

Warrior's Society of the Santa Ana Mountains
(Mountain bike advocacy group for the Cleveland National Forest)
www.warriorssociety.org

Appendix C: If you need general information about mountain biking areas . . .

Angeles National Forest
www.fs.fed.us/r5/angeles
701 North Santa Anita Avenue
Arcadia, CA 91006
(626) 574-5200

Bureau of Land Management, California State Office
www.blm.gov
2800 Cottage Way, Suite W-1834
Sacramento, CA 95825-1886
(916) 978-4400

Catalina Island Conservancy
www.catalinaconservancy.org
P.O. Box 2739
Avalon, CA 90704
(310) 510-1299

California State Parks
parks.ca.gov
(800) 777-0369

National Park Service, Santa Monica Mountains
www.nps.gov/samo
401 West Hillcrest Drive
Thousand Oaks, CA 91360
(805) 370-2301

Santa Monica Mountains Conservancy
smmc.ca.gov
(310) 589-3200
(323) 221-8900

Appendix D: If you need bike repairs, bike gear, bike parts, or whole bikes . . .

Cynergy
2300 Santa Monica Boulevard
Santa Monica, CA 90404
(310) 857-1500

Epic Cycles
120 North Topanga Canyon Boulevard, Suite 115
Topanga, CA 90290
(310) 455-1650

Helen's Cycles
www.helenscycles.com
Locations in Santa Monica, Westwood, Beverly Hills, Arcadia, Manhattan Beach, and
Marina Del Rey
(310) 829-1836

Michael's Bicycles
2253 Michael Drive
Newbury Park, CA 91320
(805) 498-6633

Performance Bicycles
www.performancebike.com
Locations in Santa Monica, Fountain Valley, Torrance, Pasadena, Laguna Hills,
Fountain Valley, Tustin, and Ventura
(800) 727-2433

REI
www.rei.com
Locations in Northridge, Santa Monica, Santa Ana, Arcadia, Manhattan Beach, and
Huntington Beach
(800) 426-4840

Wheel World Bicycles
www.wheelworld.com
Locations in Culver City and Woodland Hills
(800) 529-2530

Appendix E: If you're bored at work and the boss isn't looking . . .

www.mtbr.com—a great resource for trail and race info, product reviews, and other neat stuff

www.singletrackmind.com—a spectacular online trail guide for Southern California

www.socalmtb.com—a forum-based site with information on all topics of interest to Southern California mountain bikers

www.topozone.com, www.trails.com—Web sites that offer downloadable topographic maps for a small fee

Index

DEAR CUSTOMERS AND FRIENDS,

SUPPORTING YOUR INTEREST IN OUTDOOR ADVENTURE, travel, and an active lifestyle is central to our operations, from the authors we choose to the locations we detail to the way we design our books. Menasha Ridge Press was incorporated in 1982 by a group of veteran outdoorsmen and professional outfitters. For 25 years now, we've specialized in creating books that benefit the outdoors enthusiast.

Almost immediately, Menasha Ridge Press earned a reputation for revolutionizing outdoors- and travel-guidebook publishing. For such activities as canoeing, kayaking, hiking, backpacking, and mountain biking, we established new standards of quality that transformed the whole genre, resulting in outdoor-recreation guides of great sophistication and solid content. Menasha Ridge continues to be outdoor publishing's greatest innovator.

The folks at Menasha Ridge Press are as at home on a white-water river or mountain trail as they are editing a manuscript. The books we build for you are the best they can be, because we're responding to your needs. Plus, we use and depend on them ourselves.

We look forward to seeing you on the river or the trail. If you'd like to contact us directly, join in at www.trekalong.com or visit us at www.menasharidge.com. We thank you for your interest in our books and the natural world around us all.

SAFE TRAVELS,

Bob Sehlinger

BOB SEHLINGER
PUBLISHER

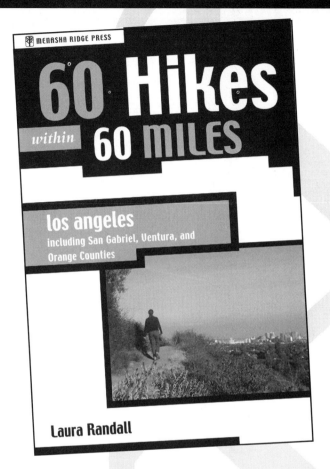

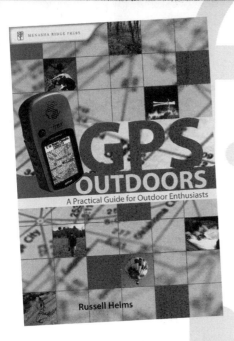
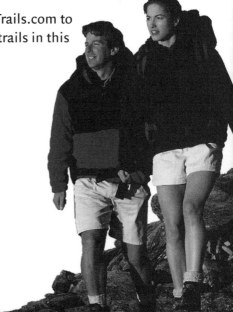
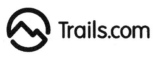